Praise for *Body Image Inside Out*

"Deb Schachter and Whitney Otto illuminate the path to transforming your relationship with body shame. Through a combination of thoughtful discussions, reflections, and exercises, *Body Image Inside Out* will help you shift from trying to push past your negative body image to regarding it as a meaningful source of information that will help you find the off-ramp from endless shame spirals. Clinicians will also appreciate this engaging, non-pathologizing workbook as a valuable resource that will facilitate their clients' healing."

Jeanne Catanzaro, Ph.D. and author of *Unburdened Eating: Healing Your Relationship with Food and Your Body Using an Internal Family* ~~~ *Approach*

"I have been in the field of eating disor~~~ ~~~ ~~~ ~~~ ~~~ ~~~ ~~~ ~~~ attest to the fact that dealing with body image is ~~~ ~~~ ~~~ ~~~ ~~~ ~~~ plicated aspects of my work. Whitney and Deb pr ~~~ ~~~ ~~~ ~~~ ~~~ ion and exercises to heal body image wounds a ~~~ ~~~ ~~~ ~~~ others turn their relationship with their bodies, ~~~ ~~~ ~~~ ~~~ ~~~ ." Both clinicians and clients can benefit from reading this book."

Carolyn Costin, MA, MEd, MFT, CEDS, FAED The Carolyn Costin Institute and Author of *The Eating Disorder Sourcebook, 8 Keys to Recovery From an Eating Disorder*

"As an Olympic athlete for almost two decades, I grounded my identity in what my body could do. Now that I am retired from competition, I face the loss of this identity. When I began reading *Body Image Inside Out*, tears rolled down my face as I realized how those feelings of loss are connected to my body. This book helped me forge a new relationship with my body and, by extension, a new identity."

Caryn Davies, 2x Olympic Champion, Founder, Podium Law, 2023 Recipient of the Thomas Keller Medal

"Deb and Whitney have written the body image book I've longed to hand to all of my clients. Through relatable vignettes and engaging exercises, they answer the illusive question, "What do I do with how badly I feel in and about my body?" Our bodies have never been the problem. And *Body Image Inside Out* shows readers that not only are our bodies not a problem to be solved but that turning towards our negative body image has the power to reveal what we most need to know about ourselves. If you have ever struggled with your body image, there's something in this book for you."

Marci Evans, MS, RDN, LDN Food and Body Image Healers®

"At last, an inspiring, provocative and effective guide for how to love and respect our bodies and ourselves. This superbly friendly, well-written book gives real muscle to the process of healing a loveless marriage with our bodies that many of us find ourselves in. The stories and exercises dance off the page with effortless ease, making real, tangible change feel not only possible but joyful, happening moment by moment as you read. Liberating and powerful, this is the best, most practical book about body image I have come across."

Claire Dale, Founder/Director Physical Intelligence Institute, Author of the award-winning book *Physical Intelligence*

"This book provides a much-needed resource for helping heal body image. Using vivid real-world cases and practical exercises, *Body Image Inside Out* convincingly and compassionately shows that body image challenges have more to do with our relational life and emotional circumstances than they do with the actual body we find ourselves in. Readers will find this to be a deeply healing experience. I will be recommending this wonderful book to many of my patients!"

Jennifer L. Gaudiani, MD, CEDS-C, FAED, Founder & Medical Director of the Gaudiani Clinic and Author of *Sick Enough: A Guide to the Medical Complications of Eating Disorders*

"I wish I could jump in a sporty time machine and give this book to my teenage self. Grateful to be reading it now! If you've had it with being an enemy (or frenemy) of your body, read this book!"

Amanda Hennessey, Public Speaking Coach, Actress and Author of *Your Guide to Public Speaking*

"How we see ourselves indeed changes everything and I am in awe of the depth and importance of the wisdom in this book. I have never before explored how my body image could become a living, daily prompt for me to more deeply understand myself and my story. I have never before considered my body image as a hero.

Body Image Inside Out is full of powerful, clarifying and diverse stories that informed and inspired me to see how body image + curiosity + compassion + connection can be a formula for powerful healing and change . . . in both ourselves and the world. This book took my understanding of the profound intelligence that lives in our bodies to another level. I will return to these potent questions and exercises again and again and am already looking in the mirror and walking through the world differently because of what I learned."

Cara Jones, Coach, Storyteller, *Untethered Voice* Podcast Host

"*Body Image Inside Out* will help you dive deep into your body image story while acting as a compassionate guide toward decoding body peace. I wish I had this resource years ago."

Leslie Schilling, RD and Author of *Feed Yourself*

"In 20 years of working with women, I've never met one who hasn't spent hours, months, years or decades grappling with and lamenting her body image. Of all the relationships a woman must navigate in a misogynist culture, it is the relationship to her body image that is perhaps the most complicated, confusing and confronting.

Body Image Inside Out is a powerful and practical guide for flipping the paradigm of body-as-enemy to body as an intelligent ally and vessel of wisdom.

A must read for every woman, every feminist and every body."

Megan Jo Wilson, Founder, Rockstar Camp for Women

"As an Olympic athlete I was rewarded for pushing my body past my physical and mental limits. I had to learn that my body is not just a vehicle for my goals. This insightful book offers a brand new and heart centered perspective on how to build friendship and connection with one's body, and how to tap into its wisdom."

Iris Zimmermann, US Olympic Fencer, Executive Coach, *Untrained* Podcast Co-host

Body Image Inside Out

A Revolutionary Approach to Body Image Healing

Deb Schachter MSW &
Whitney Otto MA, PCC

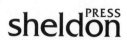
sheldon PRESS

First published by Sheldon Press in 2024
An imprint of John Murray Press

1

A CIP catalogue record for this title is available from the British Library

Trade Paperback ISBN 9781399816212
ebook ISBN 9781399816205

Library of Congress Control Number: 2024934079

Typeset by KnowledgeWorks Global Ltd.

Printed and bound in the United States of America

John Murray Press policy is to use papers that are natural, renewable and recyclable products and made from wood grown in sustainable forests. The logging and manufacturing processes are expected to conform to the environmental regulations of the country of origin.

John Murray Press
Carmelite House
50 Victoria Embankment
London EC4Y 0DZ

www.sheldonpress.co.uk

John Murray Press, part of Hodder & Stoughton Limited
An Hachette UK company

There are places in all of us that have been measured, ignored or shamed. This book is dedicated to the healing we believe is possible when we learn to listen to them.

Contents

About the Authors

Whitney Ladd Otto, MA, PCC, is a certified coach and group facilitator with over three decades of experience in leadership development, high performance and personal transformation. She co-hosts the podcast, *Untrained*, offering compassionate and innovative strategies for achieving sustainable high performance. Whitney's personal journey towards deeper embodiment has profoundly shaped her professional approach, enabling her to appreciate and harness the inherent wisdom of the body in her work. She lives in Cambridge, Massachusetts, with her husband, a psychology professor, and their daughter and son.

As a pioneer in the field of body image, **Deb Schachter, LICSW,** has dedicated her 30-year career to helping people unpack their body's story and the wisdom it has to offer. Blending together her West Coast spirit and her East Coast sensibility, her work is grounded in the power of connection. Deb facilitates multiple ongoing body image and recovery groups, emphasizing the insight and healing that can be accessed through courage and curiosity.

Beyond her private practice, Deb trains therapists and other health professionals, sharing her paradigm-shifting perspectives on body image and eating disorder recovery. When not BodySelfing, she enjoys creating colorful things and spending time with her favorite people and plants. She lives in Boston, MA, with her husband Jim and her spunky Goldendoodle, Soleil.

Authors' Note

Language

As authors of a book about body image, we want to address the highly charged word, "fat." The word "fat" is so often used pejoratively to discriminate, stigmatize and criticize. We do not want to add to the negative associations of this word, yet we can't change what we can't talk about. We want to explore the word "fat" for the sake of helping people uncouple negative emotions and sensations from the word. We have to name the harmful and internalized messages associated with "fat" in order to make them visible. Once these internalized messages are conscious, we can offer new ways of relating to the emotional and sensory experiences that are so often blended with the label of "fat."

While we focus on the internal experience of "feeling fat," we want to acknowledge that there are external realities facing people in larger bodies: biased medical care, seating that doesn't accommodate all bodies and cruel body commentary to name a few. We realize that no degree of internal body image work will alter the external world's anti-fat bias. What we are hoping to do in this book is to create language and strategies for people in all bodies to feel that our bodies are a safe place to inhabit.

Privilege

Body image struggles impact people of all genders, races, abilities, sizes and backgrounds. Our intention is to contribute resources to provide healing for body image. We want to acknowledge the limitations of our own perspectives. As white, cis-gendered, able-bodied straight women, we recognize the privilege we hold in navigating the world and the messages we receive about our bodies. This background undoubtedly influences our experiences and therefore our work. We honor that our perspectives and exercises may not resonate with or apply to all individuals.

Foreword

The Beginning

People often ask us, "What does it mean to specialize in body image?" "What do you actually do?" "Can people really improve their body image and if so, how?" This book is our answer. It is filled with many people's stories, but we are going to start with the one that lies at the heart of the BodySelf philosophy: the story of *Fat Temp* (please see Authors' Note) and *Crazy Raisin*. This story reveals the qualities that we hope this book embodies: connection, curiosity and compassion.

Almost 20 years ago, a bright-eyed young woman, who recently finished her Master's degree in mental health counseling, sought out a well-known psychotherapist who specialized in eating disorders and body image for an informational interview. This recent graduate was interested in focusing on these professional areas herself and wanted to learn more. The psychotherapist found her to be earnest and energetic and her curious spirit inspiring.

If you haven't guessed it yet, this is our story ...

We, Whitney and Deb, became fast friends, bonding over our mutual love of art and the outdoors, and the deep passion we shared for healing work, both inside ourselves and with our clients. We talked about our own eating disorder recoveries and our ongoing pursuit of an easier relationship with our bodies. As our friendship deepened, we discovered that we were developing our own language for talking about body image.

Because of the safety of our friendship, we were able to expand our body image lens from the well-worn paths of shame and judgment to an open, more lighthearted frame that had been impossible to access on our own. By borrowing one another's curiosity and compassion and directing them towards the critical parts of ourselves, we created a new perspective on our negative body image. We weren't just talking about body image anymore, but the interconnected relationship *between* our stories, both past and present, and the way we felt about our bodies.

We realized what we had been calling "body image" was a multi-dimensional experience. We discovered that our body image was not just about our size or what we saw in the mirror, but actually influenced by what we came to call the BodySelf: our stories, our traumas, our temperament, our longings and our desires. We found that by developing a relationship with our BodySelves, we were moving the dial on our body image work in ways we never thought was possible.

Over time, we started to weave this new language and way of thinking into our clinical work. It resonated so much with our clients that we decided to create

BodySelf workshops, to change the conversation people were having about body image, from one of shame and suffering to one of discovery and freedom.

Meanwhile, we continued on our own BodySelf journeys, and developed a habit of giving endearing names to our various body image self-perceptions. Creating identities for our negative body image thoughts brought a lighthearted acceptance to our most vulnerable body image beliefs, leading us to feel less ashamed of the harsh ways we saw ourselves. We came to especially appreciate two of these characters, Fat Temp and Crazy Raisin.

Fat Temp

Two years after returning from the Olympics as an alternate for the US Women's Lightweight Rowing team, Whitney sat in the basement of a university financial service department, working as a temp. While she felt some relief at having a task with a beginning, an end and a paycheck, her overall spirits were quite low. In her mind, her Olympic dream had failed, as had her marriage to another rower which had ended after only one year. Not only that, while her work consulting college athletic teams was energizing, it didn't pay the bills. She felt lost, defeated, and, as usual, fat.

On the outside Whitney presented as confident and energetic with a bio that reflected a great education and impressive athletic accomplishments. Her supervisor came down to her small, dimly lit office cubicle one day to check on her progress. He put his hands in his pockets and rocked back on his heels. "Why are you here?" he asked gently. Clearly, he didn't know how her resume had led her to this particular job in this particular basement. If she had added a line on her resume that stated, "spent a long time reeling and healing from an entrenched eating disorder and a divorce, looking for something stable and predictable with a paycheck," perhaps it might have made more sense to him.

Even though Whitney knew taking this temp job was a positive step for a variety of emotional and practical reasons, she felt great shame about it. Her body communicated its shame through a raw self-consciousness and a desire for physical change. Being at peak fitness and the intense training that supported that goal had been a huge part of her life and identity for a long time. She had also been a "lightweight rower," so she was constantly comparing her current body to a weight and fitness level that used to be a full-time endeavor. Now, as she transitioned out of her rowing career, these unattainable goals served as an orienting focus that temporarily freed her from feelings of grief and confusion. The one-two punch of feeling "fat" and ashamed about her temp status helped distract her from looking at the bigger issues: the loss of her rowing career and marriage and the overwhelming uncertainty about how to move through the world without these anchors. Focusing on her body and weight loss gave her direction and created a simple pathway to gain a sense of control, distracting her from these daunting life questions.

Whitney called Deb to talk about the conversation with her boss. At the time, she felt like she was best summed up as someone who had just had her "15 minutes of fame" as an alternate in the Olympics and despite all her privilege and hard work, was unable to reach her potential. Together, through giggles, they named that confused and sad young woman in the basement, "Fat Temp."

Seen through Deb's eyes, "Fat Temp" was a loveable hero in transition. With Deb, Whitney could cry about how Fat Temp felt like a big failure. With Deb's compassionate reframing, Whitney's shame abated and she realized her feelings of disorientation and loss were getting redirected into her feelings about her body. She felt much more clarity about why she wanted a simple job with simple tasks and recognized, as the title implied, it was temporary.

Crazy Raisin

Meanwhile on the other side of town, Deb was 35, single, and watching her friends get engaged and married. Fresh from a breakup, Deb felt further away than ever from finding her life partner. She was committed to finding the right match and took dating very seriously. After a parade of laughably mismatched blind dates set up by friends, she waded into the online dating pool. It was crazy-making. Long text-only relationships that led to nowhere, great first dates that faded into oblivion and far too many coffee dates that had no spark. She felt like she couldn't do it anymore, that her heart didn't have the fortitude to tolerate the ups and downs of the dating world.

At the same time, Deb started noticing ways that both her body and face were aging. Having grown up as a suntanned California girl, she observed the little creases at the edge of her eyes that she swore hadn't been there the month before. Aware of the sun's impact on her skin, she put on a hat and slathered herself in sunscreen. She felt pasty, pale and disconnected from her old self. She was trying so hard to do the right things with her skin and men, and yet she still felt like she was shriveling like a raisin.

After each ridiculously incompatible date or "mini-relationship," Deb would call Whitney, feeling discouraged, hopeless and a million miles from sexy. She'd find herself wondering, "Am I crazy, or are they?" They affectionately named this part of Deb, "Crazy Raisin." Through Whitney's eyes, Deb was a highly successful, independent, youthful woman bravely searching for what she really wanted and having a hard time finding it. Together they realized that it felt easier for Deb to worry about her wrinkles and her aging body than it did to feel the confusion, vulnerability and fear surrounding her search for a partner. By recognizing the ways that Deb was channeling her angst about dating into her body image, it was her heart rather than her skin that needed her attention.

The BodySelf Workshops

Time and time again, we offered one another safety and neutrality to explore our self-hating and negative body image thoughts, creating a new mirror for one another unlike any we had before. These experiences inspired us to design exercises, prompts and tools to share the BodySelf perspective. Our first workshops took place in Deb's office, where 18 people crammed into a room built for 8. As attendance grew, we became more adventurous and held the workshops in borrowed yoga and tai chi studios, YMCA event rooms (once with a spirited African drumming session going on next door), church basements and college classrooms. In these rooms, we continued to hone the BodySelf approach and the best ways to help participants develop a relationship *with* their body image.

We saw eyes light up, shoulders relax and conversations kindle as attendees realized that there was so much more to talk about than how much they hated their bodies. Shame was swapped out for curiosity, connections were made internally and externally, and the daily, relentless negativity about their bodies started to shift. Participants now had a language and a framework for how to be in relationship with their bodies in a new way. They were relieved to find out that the BodySelf approach didn't require them to dance like a leaf, stand naked in front of a mirror or feel like they should let go of wanting to feel beautiful and powerful in their bodies. Instead of encouraging people to reject negative body image, the workshops gave them permission to lean into it, giving them the ability to translate the language of their body image into valuable information about themselves and the kinds of lives that they wanted to lead. Conversations that began with a focus on stomachs, butts and thighs evolved into dialogues about self-expression, grief, passion, trauma and the pursuit of a more satisfying and aligned life.

After two decades of seeing the BodySelf approach help people transcend the glass ceiling of negative body image, we wanted to expand the reach of our message.

*At the end of each chapter you will find a blessing.
John O'Donahue describes a blessing as 'a circle
of light' that is drawn around a person to
strengthen, protect and heal.*

*The chapters in this book are designed to help you free
yourself from negative body image patterns, and the
blessings were created to solidify the teachings within
you. Their purpose is to encircle you with new and
kinder opportunities for being in relationship with
your body and body image.*

1 | Welcome to the Conversation

"Curiosity is an act of vulnerability and courage. We need to be brave enough to want to know more."

Brené Brown

Welcome—It Takes Courage to Be Here!

We imagine you opened this book because you or someone you love is sad, frustrated or tired from a battle with their body image. We get it. We have been having honest conversations with people about body image for decades. Everyone has a story, though rarely has it been shared, because most people don't have safe spaces or the right language to talk about body image. People long for more freedom and body acceptance but are also frightened to let go of the mental attachments and ideals that we associate with having "the right body."

We are well-trained to criticize our bodies and talk about what we'd like to change. Rarely are we taught to bring curiosity to the experience of living in our bodies and the way we see ourselves. In this book, we want to help you deconstruct the messages and experiences that have influenced your own body image "story." We wrote this book to help you build a relationship between you and your body image through tools that offer more freedom and connection. We think of our work as a type of couples therapy for you and your body image.

We are glad you are here. In showing up, you are acknowledging that you want more ease in the relationship you have with your body. We are offering a new perspective on relating to your body rather than trying to "fix it." We promise that we will not ask you to celebrate your favorite body part or declare love for your body while wearing a burlap sack. Nor will we promise that you will wake up every day loving your body fully if only you follow our process. Instead, we will offer you practical and creative tools like:

- How to understand and shift your habitual body image thoughts and behaviors.
- How to decode what it is you really want from that "fix my body" plan you are considering.
- How to use your jealousy as a teacher rather than a tormentor.

- How to identify which relationships trigger your negative body image and how to respond differently.
- How to prepare for bad body image days so that when they show up, you can resource and connect rather than hate and ignore.

What the Heck is Body Image, Really?

Body image can be defined as the subjective picture or mental image of one's own body. But where does this subjective image come from? We each have a unique story of how we see ourselves and how we believe we are seen. This internalized image is a composite of our experiences: all the messages and beliefs that we have taken in about ourselves and our bodies, and perhaps most importantly, how these experiences get held, processed and expressed through our bodies. Body image can have so many functions: as a companion, a distraction, a resource for control and a perceived vehicle for hope. Each offering us the promise of greater love and acceptance if we get our bodies "right."

Is Our Body Image Separate from Our Body?

How we see ourselves can be very different from the physical form of our bodies. Body perception and body form can influence one another, but they are separate. Body shape and size shift over weeks, months and years; body perceptions can change on a dime. They are influenced by multiple factors: our histories, moods, life stressors, relationships, disappointments, achievements, food choices, exercise, weather and hormones, to name a few. What we perceive in the mirror is often not informed by a fixed external reality but by these factors that are forever in flux.

Is Fat a Feeling?

We get this question a lot and it's a complex one to answer. Fat is an adjective, just like tall, freckled or strong. In this book we are going to talk about how the perceived experience of "feeling fat" has become shorthand for complex emotions and the sensations that accompany them. We are going to dig into the idea that how you feel *in* your body can become how you feel *about* your body. For example, "I feel so full of feelings" can quickly morph into feeling "fat" with feelings. How many times have you said to yourself, "I feel badly about my body" when it would have been more accurate to say, "I feel sad, lonely, confused or hopeless and it just feels like too much." When we invite our clients to explore what "fat" means to them through words or art, we end up with vastly different language, colors and shapes. The way we describe our bodies holds a world of meaning and learning to decode that deeper meaning is what this book is all about. To answer the original question, fat isn't a feeling, yet the word can be a portal to sensations, feelings and emotions unique to each person.

Why Do I Spend So Much Time Hating My Body?

Negative thoughts about our body offer us a bridge between pain and hope, a way to shift from the discomfort of the present moment towards a hope for what we think we will receive if we change our body. Negative body image can be a proxy or stand-in for painful or unsatisfying aspects of our ongoing experiences and a receptacle for our unprocessed feelings, such as fear, anger, hurt or disappointment. Focusing on our bodies gives us an illusion of having control over aspects of our lives where we are suffering. Even if the voice of our negative body image is our constant critic, it can become a way to feel safe and oriented. Focusing on our body offers us a roadmap when other aspects of our life don't make sense. In short, having the "right" body is mistakenly seen as a gateway to more life satisfaction and connection and this pursuit is hopeful ... and endless.

Why is a Focus on Improving Your Body So Compelling?

A body image focus can provide a "container" of sorts for life's messier elements. When life is disappointing, a body image focus provides a place to "house" our unmet needs and desires. When life gets complex, a body image focus provides simplicity. When emotions are overwhelming, a body image focus offers a plan and a sense of control. When our important relationships are lacking in connection and safety, a body image focus provides an explanation for this emotional distance as well as a perceived path for reconnection. In the short term, focusing on changing our body is a compelling strategy, providing a platform for emotional regulation. Yet over time, a body image focus moves us further away from what we truly long for and need.

How Does Negative Body Image Develop?

Negative body image is something that is constructed over time and can be a combination of many influences:

- How much we felt seen, understood and cared for in our family systems and broader cultures.
- Whether it was safe to express our feelings and how well (or not) we were taught to navigate them.
- Ways that our negative body image tries to hold, manage or "contain" unprocessed hurts, losses and needs.

- What key figures in our life reflected to us about our bodies and how that made us feel.
- The belief that by improving and changing our appearance, we will gain more acceptance and connection.

What Role Does Diet Culture Play in Fostering Body Image Discontent?

As we know well, there is a multi-billion-dollar industry that promotes self-improvement by changing our bodies: surgeries, weight-loss supplements, cleanses, keto, paleo, gluten free or intermittent fasting. The language surrounding body transformation is often extreme, inaccurate and unsafe. Every day there are more workouts, apps and diets available to us, none of which take into account what is happening underneath the desire to change our bodies. Rarely is there a focus on, or curiosity about, what we hope to achieve *inside* with the diet or exercise program. We aren't trained to ask ourselves questions like, "What do I actually think will be different if I can fit into this bikini?" or "If I am the guy who can bench press my bodyweight, what else am I imagining will come with that?" Instead there is a steadfast assumption that becoming more fit, lean and beautiful will magically lead to more bliss and less suffering. We want to move away from this "fix it" approach and ask, what are these longings to change our body tending to and why?

What Is the Difference Between Body Image Work and Eating Disorder Recovery?

Eating disorder recovery focuses on the ways we may have used our body as a tool to try and manage our emotions and regulate our nervous systems. It is physical, emotional and mental work. Body image work is focused on the mental and emotional elements of how we see ourselves. Many people feel that even when they have experienced significant healing and recovery from an eating disorder, their negative body image continues to haunt them. While their health and recovery may be stable, it can feel like there is a glass ceiling to their body image healing.

Why Do I Feel So Much Shame When I Think About My Body Image?

One of the ironies of body image work is that while there is a cultural norm to criticize our bodies, people often feel great shame about the fact that they are so self-critical. Shame complicates body image work because we want to hide that which makes us feel ashamed. Shame is part of what gives negative body image its staying power, because it leads people to keep negative body image thoughts to themselves. It's so "normal" for people to talk about how much they ate over the holidays and how terrible they feel about it or what new diet or workout routine they are trying, but there are so few spaces where it feels safe to talk about body image in an authentic, curious and connected way.

Many people also feel confused that their body image focus feels so out of alignment with their values. We often hear things like, "I don't know why I think about my body so much, it is so superficial!" and "This shouldn't matter this much, why can't I just get over it?" People don't always identify appearance as a strong value, yet they spend a lot of time and energy evaluating themselves from that perspective.

We live in a shame-driven culture that teaches us to feel at fault for not achieving the prescribed ideals or the body we are taught to covet. And in body image work, shame can hit you from multiple angles. It shows up within our core issues, in our failure to achieve the body we have been taught to seek and in our judgment about how much space this body quest takes up. In the pages ahead, we will teach you how to relate to your body image differently and invite you to move toward it.

How Do I Start Approaching My Body Image in a New Way?

We believe that curiosity is a powerful tool in body image work. When we get critical and move into "fix it" mode, it narrows our focus. When we get curious, it widens our perspective and offers more spaciousness and choice.

Curiosity moves us from:

* "Damn it, I stopped working out for two days and my ass is bigger, I can feel it!" *to* "Wow, I am really uncomfortable; I took two days off from the gym because I was sick and now I feel huge. I wonder what is fueling that feeling?"
* "I hate how I look in this new shirt, my arms look disgusting in it" *to* "Huh, I got this shirt less than a week ago and loved it, and today looking in the mirror I hate how my arms look in it. I wonder what has changed? Why do I feel so much more critical now than I did a week ago?"

> *"My mind is a bad neighborhood I try not to go into alone."*
>
> Anne Lammott

What is the BodySelf?

The BodySelf is an approach designed to help us shift from the punitive fixing mindset to one of curiosity about what our body image is trying to communicate. It asks questions about how our body image may have offered a way to resolve hurts or taken the "hit" when there was nowhere else for our pain to go. The answers to these questions can provide us with powerful information about where our healing needs to be directed.

Many assume that the goal of body image work is to distract, redirect and move away from the negative thoughts, the comparing and the self-evaluation, with the hope that by focusing on the positive aspects of ourselves, these thoughts and feelings will shrink and, over time, disappear. We believe that it is by turning towards our negative thoughts, not away, that we will find the deeper body image freedom that we crave.

The BodySelf approach offers a unique way to explore the connections between our emotional life and our experiences of our body image. It challenges the belief that by changing our bodies, we can change our lives. It views negative body image as a portal to our embodied experiences. It turns body image *inside out* and explores the stories our bodies hold and what these stories have to teach us. We believe that body image work is learning to shift from: "what is my negative body image saying *about* me?" to "what is my body image saying *to* me?"

Is BodySelf a Noun or a Verb?

Much like words such as *love*, *light* or *poop*, BodySelf is a noun and a verb.

BodySelf [body self]

noun

1. An approach and practice that explores how negative body image beliefs are shaped by our environment, history, culture and the context of the present moment. It is a framework to investigate and heal negative body image through a lens of mindful awareness, curiosity and compassion.

Usage: *Have you heard about that cool new book about how to get in touch with your BodySelf?*

verb

2. The act of exploring, relating to and healing one's negative body image through a framework of mindful awareness, curiosity and compassion.

Usage: *You sound awfully critical of your body, you might want to do some BodySelfing.*

How to Use This Book: The BodySelf Way

Body image negativity is an individual sport, trained in isolation. The grand paradox is that the ultimate goal of improving our body image is motivated by a desire for greater connection with others (adoration, desirability, acceptance, etc.) yet the path to get there almost always keeps us more alone. People want more connection but the fix-your-body path is often profoundly lonely. Starving ourselves makes us feel anti-social, being obsessive keeps us in our head and over-exercising can lead us to miss out on social plans. We believe there is healing in the simple act of coming together and sharing: realizing we are not alone and there is another way. We have found that the thoughts that feel dreadful when we are at home alone trying on ten pairs of jeans, can make us laugh when we share the story with other people who have had similar experiences. Negative body image is created in isolation and healed through connection. This book is a gateway to start to build your body image connections.

For many of you, this might be your first "body image work" rodeo and it may feel safest to start by exploring the chapters and exercises on your own. We hope that while you may be reading this book by yourself, you might feel a bit less alone with your body image struggles. We want to help you bring more awareness, curiosity and healing to these internal body image conversations. The BodySelf approach is rooted in the belief that connection amplifies healing. We have had first-hand experience that we all hold an innate and powerful ability to heal through the act of being seen and witnessing one another.

We also want to encourage people to have these conversations in community. One of the best ways to heal is to "borrow" compassion and non-judgment from others while cultivating it in yourself. Talking about body image in safe spaces helps people feel less ashamed and more compassionate and connected. So, if you have the opportunity to read this book with others, we cheer you on. And, if you are not yet quite ready to share your body image journey, honor that instinct, take your time and share your thoughts, feelings and discoveries with people you trust when you are ready.

Compassion Caveat

The exercises in each chapter can be enlightening *and* emotionally provocative. Before you jump into each one, look them over. There will likely be tender and vulnerable phases during your body image journey, so approach this book in whatever way feels right to you.

You may also want to be intentional about where and when you do these exercises. What kind of space might feel right? What might feel supportive to your body, physically and emotionally? Take a moment to think about what might feel good: a blanket on your lap or background music. Think about what time of day might feel best, giving yourself the emotional space you need.

Exercise 1.1 Starting the Conversation: Some Questions to Answer

Why did you pick up this book? Or why do you think someone gave it to you or recommended it?

What are you most curious to learn about? What do you want more of in your life that might be gained by feeling freer in your own skin?

Are there aspects of living in your body that offer you ease or peace?

Exercise 1.2 Create Your Own Body Image Cluster

One of the first exercises we always do at the beginning of our workshops is to "cluster" body image. It's like your own individual map of what body image means to you in this moment and what it might have to tell you. It's an exercise that might look different every time you do it.

You will see "body image" written in the center of the square image below. What is the first thing you think of when you see "body image?" Write that down. Write down more words you associate with "body image." Then write down any words associated with those words. Keep going until you fill the page or you feel like you are done. Now take a look at all the words on the page. What do you notice about what you see? Any themes emerge?

This cluster will help you start to explore your associations with body image.

Example:

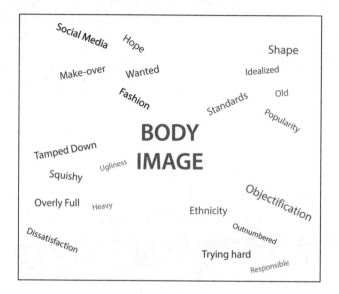

Your Turn:

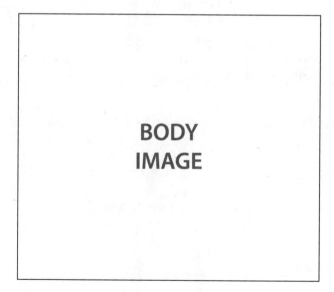

Exercise 1.3 Embodied Cluster (example below)

Pick the word/s that stand out to you in your cluster, the ones that have the most "charge" for you, that evoke a strong emotional response. Now look at the figure below and see if there is a place on the body that you feel that word should go. Perhaps close your eyes for a moment and see if you have a sense of where the word feels like it might live *in* or *on* your body. It can be how you feel about a part of your body or it can also be where the thought lives in your body. Or it might just be that the word belongs somewhere and you aren't sure why.

My words are: _____

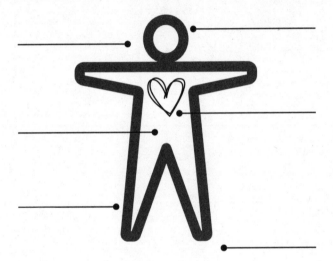

Example:

My words are: Responsible, Squishy, Heavy, Overly full, Tamped down

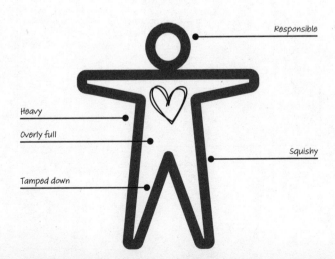

Exercise 1.4 Mindset Check-in

We want to capture your current body image mindset. This will help clarify your starting point on your BodySelf journey. You will get the chance to do this again in Chapter 10 so that you can compare the two.

My current body image mindset (example below):

What I believe to be true about my body image is:

_____

_____

The way this makes me feel is:

_____

_____

The way this makes me act is:

_____

_____

The way I want to feel is:

_____

_____

The way I want to act is:

_____

_____

Example:

What I believe to be true about my negative body image is:

It's something I don't have any control over.

The way this makes me feel is:

Discouraged, frustrated and worn out.

The way this makes me act is:

I spend more time than I want trying to figure what to wear. I often cancel plans because I feel so crummy in my body.

The way I want to feel is:

Free and more confident.

The way I want to act:

To have more fun getting dressed and to have how I feel about my body not hold me back from doing things I want to do.

Bless these bodies, our faithful companions.

*Bless this process of starting a
new relationship with them.*

*May we relax into the enoughness of
our bodies in this moment.*

*May we invite compassion into our stories and
explore them from new perspectives.*

Bless whatever truth wants to be born.

*Bless our bodies, and all that they know
and have to teach us.*

2 | Embracing the BodySelf

"We can't solve problems by using the same kind of thinking we used when we created them."

Albert Einstein

I Don't Want to Talk About It

We have been facilitating groups and workshops for over twenty years and we are still amazed by what happens when we first start to talk about body image. It is a whole-body event. People's postures change as they curl into themselves: gazes drop down, hands clasp elbows and knees pull tightly together. Typically, talking about body image triggers uncomfortable thoughts, beliefs and emotions. Most people fear that if they turn inward toward these negative body thoughts, they will feel much worse. They assume that their body image is something to manage, fix or change. The BodySelf approach introduces the idea that our body image is something to get to know and ultimately to build a healthy relationship with.

Moving Away from A One-Dimensional Image

The factors that influence how we see ourselves are complex. By the time we reach young adulthood, we have been exposed to millions of images of idealized bodies. Although we have been socialized to think that what we see in the mirror is who we are, body image is actually a multi-dimensional experience. Body image is fluid rather than static and shifts in response to our internal and external environments. Have you ever felt solid about your body in the morning, only to return home after a rotten day to criticize what you see in the mirror? Or on the flip side, have you ever felt pretty "meh" about how you look entering your day and something shifts and suddenly you feel like you look pretty damn good? A body image boost could come from receiving great feedback at work, starting to plan a trip you have dreamed about for years or receiving a flirty response on your dating app. In contrast, your body image can tank after a dinner with a hurtful family member, having an old knee injury reappear or feeling ignored by a friend. How we see ourselves is subject to multiple factors and getting curious about these factors is at the core of building a BodySelf experience. We need to delve deeper than the image and turn our focus inside out to discover what is going on.

So … What Is the BodySelf Experience?

While the images you see in magazines, on billboards and on your phone are two-dimensional, the BodySelf experience is multi-dimensional and inside of you. It holds your history, beliefs, dreams and fears. The BodySelf tools help interpret the stories each of our bodies has to tell. The BodySelf approach invites you to access the layers of lived experiences and longings in *your* unique body.

The BodySelf Mindset

- Body image is fluid and influenced by many factors, both past and present.
- We can move from "I don't like what I see," to "What is going on inside that might be affecting the way I see myself?"
- Rather than looking at poor body image as a pathology, we can see it as a gateway to greater alignment with ourselves.
- We don't have to change our physical body to change our body image.

"The wound is the place where the light gets in."

Rumi

Listening to Body Image

Sometimes it feels like our body image has a megaphone and is screaming in our ears about our imperfections. We want to help you ask your negative body image to put down that megaphone and step forward for a conversation using an indoor voice. When the volume of that critical voice is turned down, and we can bring more curiosity to how we are talking to ourselves about our body, other valuable information can come through. For example, exploring the emotions around the mundane yet sometimes loaded practice of getting dressed or packing for a trip can offer valuable insight if we ask the right questions. When we pause and bring curiosity to our struggle about what to wear or pack, it allows us to expand the moment and have access to what might otherwise be invisible.

Imagine a woman getting ready for an interview for a job she has dreamed about for years. After a rigorous graduate school education and a career with long and punishing hours, she is up for a director position at a company she believes in. Despite her impressive background and preparation, she has convinced herself that finding the right shirt to wear will make or break her ability to land the job. If she were able to slow down, she might recognize that her fixation on picking the perfect shirt is an attempt to manage all that is feeling out of her control, including succeeding as a female in a male-dominated industry.

Imagine a man getting ready for a college reunion who is feeling unusually body conscious and critical, like nothing he puts on looks right. If he were able to dig a little deeper and wonder about his struggle to pick clothes that "look good," he might recognize his feelings about being newly sober and his concern about reconnecting with his old drinking buddies without a beer in his hand.

Most people have struggled at some point in their lives, seemingly unable to find the right outfit. What if there isn't anything wrong with our clothes? What if what we are trying to manage is the vulnerable feelings that arise in the process of getting dressed? Curiosity is the portal to more insight and can help differentiate the outfit from the meaning the outfit has.

Client Spotlight: So Much More than Pants

Julia was packing for a vacation with her new girlfriend, Jessie. They were headed to Jessie's family's cabin in New Hampshire for a week and Julia was going to be meeting Jessie's parents and siblings for the first time. Initially, it seemed straightforward—a low key New Hampshire cabin vibe, right? But packing felt incredibly stressful and overwhelming. Every pair of pants Julia tried on felt too "something": too tight, too uncomfortable, too boring or just plain ugly. It felt like, somehow, overnight her body had changed and not one pair of pants felt like they fit. How did picking pants for an informal outdoorsy weekend suddenly become so impossible? When Julia was able to get curious about what was happening internally, she realized that this packing dilemma was a reminder of how many times throughout her life she had struggled to find clothing that felt right rather than gender-conforming. While Julia knew that Jessie's family had accepted that she and Jessie were a couple, it was clear from how Jessie described her coming-out experience that her parents were still very much in a process of becoming comfortable with their daughter's sexuality.

As Julia reflected on why she felt so hijacked by her search for the perfect pants, she realized that she felt like she was in a double bind. She imagined that if she brought the clothing that she felt most comfortable in—pants that felt aligned with the queer culture that she and Jessie identified with—she might make Jessie's parents uncomfortable. On the other hand, dressing in stereotypically feminine clothing would leave Julia herself feeling uncomfortable and inauthentic. The stakes felt high and the decisions felt loaded. In exploring this struggle further, Julia started to more fully appreciate how much she loved Jessie and wanted to be accepted by her family. At the same time, she was able to have more compassion for her younger self, recalling how often she had overridden her clothing preferences growing up to keep her family more comfortable. The vulnerability that surfaced during her "pants conundrum" gave Julia an opportunity to be more attuned to herself, and ultimately have an honest conversation with Jessie about how she felt.

Many of us feel like there is something "wrong" with our bodies and that they need to be different. What if our bodies don't need "fixing" but instead these beliefs are actually telling us that there is some aspect of our *lives* that is feeling misaligned, painful or even "wrong" and needs our attention.

Client Spotlight: Only an Outline of Me

Brianne was adopted as an infant and knew almost nothing about her biological parents. While Brianne had brown skin, her adoptive parents were white and had been given no information about her racial background. She and her family lived in a predominantly white, middle-class community and although there was some diversity in her school, it troubled Brianne that she didn't know her racial identity. People often asked questions about her country of origin or tried to guess her race, which left Brianne feeling awkward and ashamed. She didn't have a clear group to identify with amongst her peers of color, which left her feeling even further displaced and disconnected as an adoptee. She felt "empty, almost like there is an outline, but nothing to fill in the space."

Sports had always come easily to Brianne and by middle school she found that being a forward on the girl's soccer team was the one place she felt a sense of identity and belonging. When she transitioned from middle school to a much larger high school, the comments and questions about her race escalated. She responded by investing more time and energy into her fitness training and perfecting her body in order to compensate for feeling so unmoored socially. Her food intake and workout schedule became extremely regimented in order to pursue her star athlete status.

It wasn't until Brianne went to college and suffered a devastating sports injury, that she started therapy. The temporary loss of her fitness routine and disconnection from her sport identity opened a door to explore the ways that focusing on her body had served her. She began to understand how her intense training had been trying to manage the parts of her that had felt so undefined and out of place. She realized that pushing and perfecting her body had been a way to override her feelings of confusion, loss and disconnection. Once she was able to understand her body image story and the ways that her body focus was trying to help her, she could start to re-evaluate the intensity she brought to her athletic journey and attend to her feelings around her identity.

"Curiosity is the gentle friend that teaches us how to become ourselves."

Elizabeth Gilbert

Creating Space Between You and Your Body Image Thoughts

For most of us, there has been very little space in our mind between our thoughts *about* our bodies and the judgments that are attached *to* them. You may not have known that separating from your body image thoughts was even possible. The binary language (i.e. good/bad, fat/thin) we use to talk about our bodies can leave very little room for discovery. Bringing some awareness to how we think about our bodies uncouples the automaticity of these judgmental patterns.

When we say, *creating more space between our body and our body image*, we mean observing how we talk to ourselves *about* our body. For example, muttering under your breath "I am such a failure" every time something doesn't fit is quite different than observing that "every time something doesn't fit, I tell myself I am a failure." With this awareness, we can start to bring in curiosity to learn more about what our body image thoughts might actually be trying to communicate. This shift sounds simple yet it takes a lot of intentionality and practice. We invite you to make a shift from saying something like, "My body is disgusting, I hate my _____ [body part]" to saying, "My body image is terrible today and I am not sure why. I wonder what is making me feel so critical of myself right now?" These are two very different comments, right? In one, your sense of worth is assigned to your body image, while in the other, there is a curiosity about what feelings you might be channeling *into* your body image. What *else* might be happening that could influence how you are seeing yourself and your body?

Decoding Body Image Language

Bringing awareness to the language we use around body image can be an effective way to learn more about what is happening inside us. Let's decode things we often hear:

- "Nothing seems to fit" could mean "Will I fit in tonight?"
- "Whenever I dress for a date, I don't know what to wear" might actually be saying "Will I be able to be myself tonight? And if I am, what will happen?"
- "My _____ is too big" might translate to "Am I going to be too much for this person/group? Will they reject me?"

Client Spotlight: Betrayed by My Body

Lucia came into her therapy session describing a recent family visit that had really stirred her up. She'd had a fight with her brother that had left her hurt and angry. After describing the weekend's events and the argument that took place, she shifted her focus to the discomfort she had felt in her body at yoga that morning. "I felt huge, I didn't feel like myself. I rely on my yoga practice because I can always count on feeling calmer and more rested afterwards. But I felt like my body was getting in the way. I left feeling worse and angry that my body was betraying me."

When invited to explore the language she was using to describe her body in yoga, Lucia was able to uncover more about how the recent family visit had impacted her. She was able to see how her description of her body at her morning class—"uncomfortable, like it was getting in the way, it betrayed me"—mirrored how she had felt during the visit home: uncomfortable, in the way and betrayed. Her body was speaking for her, letting her know on a visceral level how the visit had affected her.

This realization brought Lucia to tears. Her whole life, her parents had always minimized her brother's volatile behavior toward her, repeatedly saying to Lucia, "Just get over it, you're too sensitive." They had never acknowledged how hurtful and scary it might have felt to Lucia when he was explosive. Observing her own critical body thoughts and recognizing the truths they were trying to convey, helped Lucia became clear about the impact of her visit home. Focusing on her body offered a distraction from her deeper dilemma: how could she honor her desire to spend time with her aging parents and hold a boundary with her brother? Her body hatred was trying to redirect her inner conflict into something that felt potentially "fixable."

Let's Review

- Imagine you have now entered couples therapy with your body image. It makes sense that you and your body image have developed communication patterns that are habitual and critical and leave little room for actually getting to know one another. This can change.

- How we see ourselves is influenced by much more than our external appearance. We are going to help you explore the connections between your emotional life and your experience of how you see your body.

- With more space between you and your body image, you are going to be able to learn to decode what your negative body image is saying and translate what deeper feelings and longings your negative thoughts are expressing.

> *"Including the body story along with the verbal story illuminates and awakens what has been obscured in the darkness."*
>
> Susan McConnell

Exercise 2.1 Body Image Timeline

This exercise invites you to explore your body image story and to begin the practice of bringing curiosity to your body image experience. Examining what was happening in different chapters of our lives can illuminate valuable information about our relationship with our body image. Answers to stage-specific questions about the development of a negative body image can be surprising: "It was the year my parents told us they were getting divorced," "That was when my sister got really ill and I was often alone a lot while my parents were at the hospital," "I was terrified to go to college but no one knew," or "I had a lot of changes within my friend group." Answers can also sound more like, "I don't know why I became so focused on my body at that moment. I do know that I was feeling really lonely, scared, confused, etc., and it was overwhelming."

You have important stories to tell about your unique body image journey. In that spirit, let's start to outline your experiences, by constructing your body image timeline. Give yourself permission to do this exercise at your own pace and skip any questions that don't resonate with you. The best way to do this exercise is to answer these questions in a journal or notebook so you have plenty of room to write.

Childhood:

- As a child, were you aware of your body image?
- What do you remember about what it felt like to be in your body during this time?
- What did others reflect to you about your body during this time?

- What were the significant changes in your body and how did it affect your body image?
- What other factors in your life might have impacted your thoughts about your body during this time?
- Were there any specific memories/experiences during these years that had a lasting impact on your body image?

Teen Years:

- What do you remember about what it felt like to be in your body during this time?
- What did your caregivers, classmates and relatives reflect to you about your body during this time?
- What were significant changes in your body during and after your adolescence and how did they affect your body image?
- What other factors in your life might have impacted your thoughts about your body during this time?
- Looking back, what did you appreciate most about yourself during this time (could be body or non-body related)?
- Were there any specific memories/experiences during these years that had a lasting impact on your body image?
- What resources did you rely on during this time?
- How did your body speak to you and were you able to listen?

(We invite you to write out each of these decades separately)

Twenties and Thirties:

- What do you remember about what it felt like to be in your body in your twenties and/or thirties?
- What did your friends, family and co-workers reflect to you about your body during this time?
- What were the significant changes in your body and how did it affect your body image?
- What other factors in your life might have impacted your thoughts about your body during this time?
- Looking back, what did you appreciate most about yourself during this time (could be body or non-body related)?
- Were there any specific memories/experiences during these years that had a lasting impact on your body image?
- What resources did you rely on during this time?
- How did your body speak to you and were you able to listen?

(We invite you to write out each of these decades separately)

Forties and Fifties:

- What do you remember about what it felt like to be in your body during this time?
- What did your friends, family and co-workers reflect to you about your body?
- What were the significant changes in your body as you approached midlife and how did it affect your body image?
- What other factors in your life might have impacted your thoughts about your body during this time?
- Looking back, what did you appreciate most about yourself during this time (could be body or non-body related)?
- Were there any specific memories/experiences during these years that had a lasting impact on your body image?
- What resources did you rely on during this time?
- How did your body speak to you and were you able to listen?

Sixties and Beyond:

- What do you remember about what it felt like to be in your body during this time?
- What did your family and friends reflect to you about your body during this time?
- What were the significant changes in your body after menopause and how did it affect your body image?
- What other factors in your life might have impacted your thoughts about your body during this time?
- Looking back, what did you appreciate most about yourself during this time (could be body or non-body related)?
- Were there any specific memories/experiences during these years that had a lasting impact on your body image?
- What resources did you rely on during this time?
- How did your body speak to you and were you able to listen?

What was it like to complete the exercise above? Is there anything that became more clear to you in examining your body image journey in this way? Chances are, this exercise might have been uncomfortable or explored aspects of your story that you may not have considered before. If so, we invite you to take a moment to honor the courage of doing this exercise and check in with your body. Perhaps get yourself some water or tea, take some deep breaths, feel your feet on the floor or take some time to stretch or move your body in ways that feel good.

Reflection:

_____

_____

_____

_____

_____

Bless the space between you and your body image.

May you notice the sharp and steely words you choose when addressing your body, and try softer, looser-fitting ones.

May you turn toward curiosity over and over until it becomes your trusted companion.

Bless the space between you and your body image ... May this space become kinder and more connected.

3 | The BodySelf Muscles

"Over time, I strengthened into a different version of myself. I had new muscles, a new way of moving through the world."

Mari Andrew

Many of us have spent years honing the fine art of comparing, criticizing and craving a specific body shape or image. And let's face it, the beauty and fitness industries invest heavily in teaching people how to do this well. Most of us need to unlearn the habit of picking ourselves apart and learn a new way of being in relationship with our bodies and our body image. Before we can decode what our body image is telling us, we need to learn how to *listen* to it with a mind that is aware, curious and compassionate. In the following sections, we are going to share these fundamental BodySelf muscles and how to strengthen them.

Muscle #1: Mindful Awareness

With all of the distractions in life and the busy pace at which most of us operate, being present to how we are feeling in the moment can be challenging. Tracking what is happening inside us is foundational to BodySelfing. This practice of observing is simultaneously simple and difficult, because we have had so many years of training to automatically respond towards ourselves with judgment. In the BodySelf process, mindful awareness provides an alternative to running on the autopilot of negative self-evaluation.

The core of mindful awareness is noticing what is happening without evaluating it. It's not just paying attention to our thoughts but our sensations, our feelings and our responses to these sensations and feelings. When we gently redirect our attention to what is happening in the moment, we can have more clarity and choice.

"Equanimity is seeing what is happening without being caught up with what we see."

Sebene Selassie

Mindful awareness moves us into the fertile territory below the polarity of good and bad, where there is more to learn and experience. It is a skill that is built over time, a habit of noticing our reactions to both mundane and stressful moments, without actively judging these reactions or changing anything about how we think or behave. It can be helpful to have a grounding practice to bring us to the present moment, such as taking a breath or feeling our feet on the ground. We can use the following guided practice to mindfully center ourselves.

Just notice ...

- What am I thinking about in this moment?
- What sensations am I aware of in this moment?
- What part of my body feels comfortable (or neutral) in this moment?
- Where am I putting my attention in this moment?
- What else may be competing for my attention in this moment?
- How am I reacting to what I am noticing? Am I having thoughts and feelings about what I notice inside?

Mindfulness tip: You might try to pair your mindful practice with something you do every day—this is called habit stacking. With habit stacking you use an existing habit as a cue to call forth a new habit. For example, you might use brushing your teeth or your morning coffee as a cue to take a deep inhale or notice your feet on the ground.

> *"Thinking is incredibly useful, it just isn't our only way of knowing."*
>
> Amanda Blake

Adding Sensations to Your Mindful Awareness

Our mind speaks in thoughts, our body speaks in sensation. Sensation is how our body communicates without edit or apology. Sensations are at the core of our experience, yet most of us have learned to ignore or misinterpret them. We are typically encouraged to use our minds to navigate the world, make decisions and overcome challenges, often discounting the deeply accurate information our body holds about our own experience.

We can listen to what our body has to say by tuning into sensation. External sensations include things like the sound of a familiar voice or the warmth of the sun on the face. Internal sensations are what we can feel happening inside our body such as the fluttering of our heart when we see our new crush or the tightening of our shoulders in response to a boss' criticism. This experience of sensing things within our bodies is called interoception and it is a great skill to hone for your BodySelf practice.

Because many of us haven't been taught how to interpret the sensations we feel *in* our bodies, we often interpret these sensations to be saying something *about* our body. Whaaaaat!? If we don't know how to interpret what we are sensing internally, we might interpret the *heaviness* we feel in our heart about moving out of the apartment we have shared with good friends as a feeling of literal *heaviness* in our body. This sensation of *heaviness* can quickly be co-opted by body image and the original meaning and value of the emotional experience is then lost.

This unconscious redirection can also happen during an uncomfortable experience or an interaction with someone who is uninterested in our perspective, opinion or truth. Our body communicates its discomfort through emotions and their accompanying sensations. We might feel squirmy in our chair, tension in our chest or a knot in our stomach: *our body is telling us something isn't feeling right.* The trick is not to mistake this sensation as evidence that something isn't right about our body.

Emotions and their corresponding sensations in the body can easily convert into negative body image thoughts and beliefs. This internal rerouting of our experience from, "I feel bad" to "I look bad" happens because many of us weren't taught to process or express our emotions and sensory experiences. When these sensations aren't tended to directly, our body can become the scapegoat—what seems impossible to feel or say gets redirected towards "fixing," "shrinking" or "tightening" our body. As a result, emotional states like sadness, anxiety or anger, and physical sensations like "full," "jittery" or "explosive," are translated into "gross," "disgusting" or "ugly." Our truth isn't always communicated through words.

Mindful attention provides an alternative to these patterns by helping us simply notice our emotions and sensations and hone our ability to accurately describe our internal experiences. To support this process, we want to offer some examples of sensations that often accompany emotional states. The goal is to practice identifying sensations before they are interpreted by our body image in negative ways.

> *"There is a voice that doesn't use words. Listen."*
>
> Rumi

Body Sensations

Tender	Energized	Depressed
aglow	electrified	tired
cozy	open	disconnected
melting	tingly	heavy
fuzzy	churny	sore
warm	spikey	small

still
soft

Scared
cold
shaky
shivery
quaking
sweaty
trembling
raw
frozen

Sad
heavy
burdened
alone
empty
puffy
weighted
liquidy
achy
dark

Vulnerable
spilling
shaky
buzzing
small
breathless
full
sensitive
bubbly

fluid
pounding
radiating
shimmery
twitchy
tingling
nervy
flittery

Anxious
edgy
flickering
choppy
weary
twisty
dizzy
fluttery
spacey
hot
jittery

Constricted
knotted
hard
solid
armored
blocked
numb
wooden
tense
thick
cool
tight

icy
heavy
hiding
draining
disappearing
dense
closed

Open-hearted
airy
soft
alive
relaxed
smooth
spacious
light
shimmery
fluid
releasing
expansive
calm
full
open
silky
rolling
vital
awake

Exercise 3.1 Practice Labeling Sensations

Now you are ready to practice listening to your sensations. Think of a recent experience. What sensations were you feeling? Here are a few examples:

Experience: I am meeting up with my friends later for a drink.
Sensations: exhilarated, energized and buzzy

Experience: I had my annual review today and it didn't go as well as I had hoped.
Sensations: clenched, closed and queasy

Experience: I checked out some open houses today even though I am not sure if I can afford to buy a house right now.
Sensations: untethered, itchy and tingly

Experience: I bought a beautiful shirt on my way home from work for my presentation next week.
Sensations: solid, tingly and electric

Now you try (as many as you would like):

Think of a recent experience:

_____

_____

What sensations were you feeling?

_____

_____

Think of a recent experience:

_____

_____

What sensations were you feeling?

_____

_____

Think of a recent experience:

_____

_____

What sensations were you feeling?

_____

_____

Practicing Non-judgment

Once you start to bring awareness to your current experience (including your sensations), notice how you are interpreting the experience. The habit of judging is one of the greatest obstacles to hearing what your body image is telling you, as it closes down the BodySelf conversation. We have all internalized messages about how we "should" live, appear and succeed. Seeing your experience without passing judgment or assigning value requires intentional focus and practice.

We are socialized to think in an all or nothing framework, yet most of our experiences are nuanced. How do we practice non-judgment with ourselves? We start to notice when we label ourselves and our body with extreme language that has a value judgment. Having a bad body image experience is a great opportunity to notice when you are wearing Judgy-McJudgy-Pants. When we say we are "bad" or "wrong" or a part of our body is "too _____," the conversation ends. But when we are interested in *how* we observe ourselves, the conversation is just beginning.

For example, the thought:

- "I am so 'bad,' I couldn't get my lazy ass to the gym like I should have," causes us to miss out on what is happening on a deeper level: *"I am bummed I didn't get to the gym and I am saying lots of nasty things to myself. The reality is, I am really tired. It took all my energy to manage a stressful meeting at work. All I have in me is a walk tonight."*

- "I ate so much crap in the lunchroom today, I am so unhealthy," keeps us from learning information that might be useful if we were more mindful of the details: *"I feel stressed and tired. My new MBA class kept me out late last night and I didn't have time to make lunch today. Given my back-to-back meetings, I had to eat what I could find in the lunchroom. I really want to cook more on the weekends, so I have some back-up options on days like these."*

- "I was so good today! I only had a salad when I went out with my friends," misses out on what else is going on: *"I ordered a salad when I was having lunch with my friends. I was really hungry, but I've been feeling body conscious with summer around the corner. I felt like I should order something 'light' when they shared nachos and a bottle of wine. I was so focused on not eating, I was distracted and missed out on much of the conversation."*

The practice of shifting from judging our body to observing our body image thoughts can be profoundly different from our habitual patterns. Try shifting from "I am" statements to "my body image is" statements. Here are a few examples:

Judging: "I am so ugly/unattractive. Why would anyone want to be around me?"
Observing: *"My body image thoughts are so negative today. It makes me feel so terrible about myself and leads me to believe that how I look will get in the way of people being interested in getting to know me at the party tonight."*

Judging: "I am so scrawny. Nobody will notice me when I go to college in the fall."
Observing: *"My negative body image thoughts are so intense today. I am making lots of nasty judgments about my size and being so critical of my body as I sign up for my classes."*

Judging: "My ass is so saggy. I hate the way it looks in all of my pants. I have the opposite of a beach butt. No one will ever find me sexy."
Observing: *"I am so focused on my ass right now. I wish I had one of those tight, bouncy butts like the women at my gym. I find myself comparing my body to others so much more when other parts of my life feel out of control."*

Bad Body Image Moments (BBIMs) and Mindful Awareness

A BBIM is our nickname for when our negative body image spikes. Because BBIMs are so often accompanied by shame, we gave them an endearing name to neutralize the emotional charge in these moments. This language opens the door for a less judgmental response and a chance to learn more about what has been triggered or why we are hurting.

BBIMs give us the opportunity to practice mindful awareness. Ideally, self-hatred and discomfort become prompts to get curious about what emotions and sensations we are actually feeling. BBIMs are a cue to practice observing rather than judging. This information sets us up well to decode our negative body image.

Exercise 3.2 Bringing Mindful Awareness to a BBIM

Let's break down your last BBIM.

When was it and what was it like?

_____

_____

Judging: Can you capture what your critical voice was saying?

Example: Everything I put on looks awful, my body is disgusting.

_____

_____

What judgmental thoughts were present?

Example: There is no way I should go to this party tonight looking this awful.

_____

_____

Now let's practice observing:

Observing: How would you describe your body image from neutrality?

Example: I am so focused on how my clothes are fitting right now, it's hard to think about anything else.

_____

_____

Are there any other observations?

Example: When I am this critical of my body I end up feeling so down that I don't want to be around anyone.

_____

_____

Now that we have an understanding of how to untangle our critical body image thoughts from accurate observations, let's proceed to the next BodySelf muscle, curiosity.

Muscle #2: Curiosity

> _"Curiosity is the gentle friend that teaches us how to become ourselves."_
>
> Elizabeth Gilbert

Curiosity, Your Greatest Body Image Ally

It's not every day that you hear someone say, "I have been feeling really curious about my body image lately." What most of us hear is some version of, "I need to fix myself" or "I need to love myself." Curiosity is at the heart of developing our BodySelves. It is the gateway to the good stuff: all of the information that has been buried under years, decades or generations of negative self-talk. Curiosity is a pivotal skill because it invites a different conversation; it moves us away from _judging_ and _fixing_ and into _exploring_ and _discovering_. When our clients say begrudgingly, "Why the #@$% do I still believe that my size determines so much in my life?" we respond with a twinkle in our eyes and say, "That is such an excellent question! Can you ask it again without the attitude?" This evokes a smile and a little more space for curiosity.

Mindful awareness opens the door and curiosity welcomes us in. Curiosity offers a gentle way to further separate from our well-worn paths of self-hatred and negativity. It allows us to see what is happening more clearly without asking us to make any changes. Years of shame and judgment limit our thinking in ways that we may not even realize. Curiosity offers new information, perspectives and options.

Turning Our Thoughts Inside Out

Curiosity invites us to take our body criticism and turn it **INSIDE OUT.** What does that even mean? Think back to that notion that people feel ashamed that their body image woes feel "superficial" or "shallow." But people's body image perceptions are not shallow at all; there is unexplored depth and dimensionality within our negative body image. Our body image thoughts are just the surface layer of our experiences. Let's learn how to explore the layers beneath.

> *"The opposite of shame is curiosity."*
>
> Richard Schwartz

Asking Why Without the Attitude

Curiosity invites us to explore what exists between us and our body image and gives us the chance to find out more about what is going on. We want you to start to practice asking this important question: *Why am I having a BBIM now?* When we understand better *why* our body image has taken center stage, we can start to discover how our body image focus is trying to help us.

Here are some examples:

Judging: "This morning I flew from a city where it was snowing to a Caribbean island for my long-awaited winter getaway. I am suddenly in shorts and a bathing suit and hate how I look. I can't believe I am finally on vacation and I am ruining it by focusing on my body."

Observing and curious: *"Damn, it was hard to go from jeans and a sweater to a bathing suit overnight! I feel so exposed and vulnerable and am having lots of negative thoughts about my body. My jaw is clenched and my stomach feels knotted. What else is hard for me about being here? I wonder why I feel so awful."*

Judging: "This week I feel like I am spilling out of my clothes. I am sure I have gained weight. I am disgusting."

Observing and curious: *"I feel so uncomfortable in my skin, even though there is no physical reason for this change. It feels suffocating. I wonder if something in my life right now is leading me to feel this way in my body?"*

In the first statement, judgment is breathing down our neck, keeping us focused on what is wrong. In the second statement, curiosity creates more space to notice the context and wonder about what might be difficult. Feeling crappy about our body is the perfect signal to bring in curiosity. It gives us the chance to learn more about what aspect of our experience is activating our negative body image. We invite you to think of the presence of negative body image as a cue for curiosity rather than a cue to hate or fix.

> *"The ability to ask beautiful questions is one of the great disciplines of a human life."*
>
> David Perell

Beautiful Questions

Pairing observation with a question is a powerful way to practice curiosity. It might go something like this:

- "I feel overly focused on what to wear to this conference. I wonder why I am feeling so anxious about it?"
- "I have been imagining myself in a different body all week. Something shifted when I got back from my vacation. I wonder what is so hard about being home?"
- "I am dreading dinner with friends this weekend. I look awful in everything I put on. I don't always feel this way. I wonder what it is about this week that is making me feel so icky about my wardrobe and body. Or if there is something about the dinner that is activating my negative body image?"
- "I have been comparing my body to everyone on my team at work. I wonder what is going on at the office that is leading me to be so 'compare-y.'"

Exercise 3.3 Bringing Curiosity to Your BBIMs

Take your BBIM from Exercise 3.2 or feel free to chose another BBIM.

My BBIM was _____

_____

Now it is your turn to practice bringing more curiosity by pairing observation with a question. Start by observing your body image thoughts in the broader situation/context.

What I notice about the situation I was in was:

_____

_____

Example: After I went to my med school orientation, my body image got really loud.

Now let's ask a follow-up question.

What about this situation might have been hard for you?

_____

_____

Example: It feels so scary to finally be at this point in my life. I have worked so hard to get to med school. What if I can't keep up? What if I fail?

Exercise 3.4 Going on a First Date with Your Body Image

First dates are all about listening and being curious without a lot of preconceived ideas about who the other person is. What would it be like to go on a first date with your body image? We would love for you to bring that first date energy to the following questions.

In what environments do I tend to compare myself to others the most?

_____

In what season do I feel best in my body? What season is the most challenging?

_____

In which activities do I tend to have the best body image? In which do I feel the worst?

_____

What situations or experiences or tasks lead me to forget about my body image?

_____

Muscle #3: Self-compassion

"Self-compassion is the greatest regulator of all, without it your nervous system cannot find peace. It's your own love, forgiveness and acceptance that can … create that safety you crave."

Dani Fagan

- Mindful awareness opens the door
- Curiosity invites us in
- Compassion helps us connect with ourselves

Sometimes the only control we have over our circumstances is how much compassion we have for ourselves. A compassionate response deepens our connection with ourselves when faced with pain or stress. When added to the practices of mindful awareness and curiosity, self-compassion connects us with our bodies. It shifts us from going against ourselves to accompanying ourselves. It might seem that self-compassion would be the easiest, least effortful of the muscles to build, but it is often the hardest. It flies in the face of the training we have likely received and practiced in our "hustle" culture that teaches us to strive, push harder and fix.

The call for self-compassion might make you think of soft pillows, warm baths and comforting hugs, but for many people, the notion of self-compassion feels uncomfortable or even scary. Cultivating a self-compassion practice can elicit discomfort because it counters what many of us have been taught and most of us haven't been encouraged to think of as a resource when things go to shit. Extending a warm and accepting presence towards our suffering takes practice and patience.

Self-compassion is one of those words that gets thrown around a lot and yet most of us haven't gotten much instruction in how to build a self-compassion practice. At its core, self-compassion is about recognizing our suffering, knowing we are not alone in it and approaching ourselves with kindness and understanding. It's a way to validate our own experience and create more safety and connection.

"May I look at myself with the eyes of understanding and love."

Thich Nhat Hanh

A lot of people feel intimidated about how to do self-compassion "right." What does it look like to practice compassion? Here is an example:

Client Spotlight: Compassion Reframe

Catelina was helping her daughter shop for new school clothes. She was having a fun time interacting with her daughter and just before they left, she dashed into a store to try on something for herself. She picked out a cream-colored blazer, hoping it would help her feel stylish, professional and confident, but it had the opposite effect. It was tight in all the wrong places and the light color washed her out. Her morale immediately plummeted and the drive home felt like a parenting performance as she tried to hide her bad mood. Once she got home, she went into her room for some quiet and had a talk with herself. "I'm sorry you feel so awful, Catelina—I know how those lousy mirror moments can sometimes send you spiraling into negative thoughts. There is a lot going on with your aging parents and big responsibilities at work and I know sometimes looking older can really get you down. It makes sense that you feel sad and overwhelmed in this moment. Why don't you take a shower, watch a show with your daughter, go to bed early and choose an outfit you feel good in tomorrow morning."

Borrowing Compassion

When we ask workshop attendees to write down their negative body image thoughts and share them aloud, their eyes grow wide with fear. When we do this same exercise and ask participants to read each other's responses aloud, they eagerly jump to it with palpable compassion and understanding. With the first prompt, shame is triggered. With the second, compassion feels easy. Borrowing compassion is a valuable strategy when you can't yet muster it yourself.

> *"I used to think that I needed to be braver and I don't think I need to be braver anymore. I need to be kinder, and I need to be more curious—and bravery comes from that."*
>
> Elizabeth Gilbert

Exercise 3.5 Compassion History

Imagine the person you felt most understood by growing up. Maybe it was a sibling, parent, family friend or coach. It might have been your favorite teacher or your best friend.

The person I felt most understood by was:

_____

They made me feel:

_____

The way I felt in my body when I was around them was:

_____

The way they responded to (or how I imagine they would) my vulnerability was:

_____

I knew they had compassion for me when they:

_____

If I could internalize 10% of this compassion for me to myself, I would:

_____

"Be kind to yourself when you have become a guest in your own head"

Morgan Harper Nichols

Exercise 3.6 Practicing Self-compassion

Let's go back to the BBIM you have been working with or feel free to pick a new one. Now that you have learned more about the factors that might be influencing your negative body image, how could you respond with more compassion?

My BBIM was:

_____

_____

Mindful Awareness: If you take the judgment out and observe from a neutral lens, what is going on during your bad body image moment?

How would you describe your body image from neutrality?

_____

_____

Curiosity: Start by observing your body image thoughts in the broader situation/context.

What I notice about the situation I was in is:

_____

_____

Now let's ask a follow-up question.

What about this situation might have been hard for you?

_____

_____

Compassion: What compassionate response might you have for a friend in this situation?

It makes so much sense that you are feeling _____ *because:*

_____

_____

Now turn that into a compassionate response towards yourself:

It makes so much sense that I am feeling _____ *because:*

_____

_____

What I wish for myself is:

_____

_____

Example:

If you take the judgment out and observe from a neutral lens, what is going on during your bad body image moment?

How would you describe your body image from neutrality?

I am so focused on how my clothes are fitting today, it's hard to think about anything else.

Start by observing your body image thoughts in the broader situation/context.

What I notice about the situation I was in was:

when I signed up for my classes, my body image got really critical and loud.

Now let's ask a follow-up question.

What about this situation might have been hard for you?

It feels so scary to finally be at this point in my life. I have worked so hard to get to med school. What if I can't keep up? What if I fail?

What compassionate response might you have for a friend in this situation?

It makes so much sense that you are feeling terrified because:

This is a really big deal and there were many bumps along the way. I have worked for years to get to this point and there is so much vulnerability in starting new things, especially when I have worked for so long to get them.

What I wish for myself is: that I take this step by step and make sure that I reach out to the people who listen well and support me.

> *"When things change inside you, things change around you."*
>
> Anonymous

Bringing It Home

If the BodySelf muscles we have been helping you build could have a conversation with negative body image, it would sound like this:

Negative Body Image says: "I hate you, fix yourself."
Mindful awareness says: *"Can you say that without the attitude?"*

Negative Body Image says: "You look terrible."
Curiosity says: *"Hmmmmm, why are you saying that to me now ... what else is going on that might be influencing how I see my body?"*

Negative Body Image says: "You suck, what is wrong with you? You need to change your body."
Compassion says: *"I'm so sorry you are suffering right now. That sounds hard. It sounds like your body image is trying to help you manage _____. What might help?*

Bless your powers of awareness as you begin to witness more and more of yourself.

May your curiosity take you down new roads in your thoughts and behaviors.

Bless your body and mind with more kindness. May you begin to see you are both on the same team.

4 | From Storing to Storying

"The longest relationship you'll ever have is with your body."

Anna Sweeney

Our Bodies House Our Stories

Our bodies have been with us for every moment of our lives. They are designed to take care of us, to keep us alive, safe and functioning, often in exceptionally challenging conditions. They are the data bank for everything we have ever experienced. They house our stories and carry our most precious and painful moments. They have taken in all that we have seen, heard, and felt and are the vessels that hold our entire histories both consciously and unconsciously. No matter what our relationship has been with our bodies, they have been with us all along the way.

We are lucky to live in a time when a multitude of disciplines are exploring the abundant connections between mind and body. We are going to offer a way of conceptualizing how our emotional experiences are often "held" in the body and managed and expressed through our negative body image. Our hope is that while you may have picked up this book thinking that your body is the villain in your story, you will begin to see your body as a loyal companion and perhaps even a hero.

- **How can our body be a hero?** Because it has been committed to trying to keep us feeling safe when we didn't have the resources to do that on our own.
- **How does it do that?** Our body stores, or "houses," elements of our unique story, what we have taken in emotionally and physically over our lifetime.
- **Why does it do that?** Because there have likely been times that we didn't have the support to help us process and metabolize what we were feeling.
- **What role does body image play?** Negative body image offers a way to manage and redirect the overwhelming experiences that we have taken in. Focusing on our negative body image offers protection through separation: rejecting the feelings by rejecting where the story is held. When something feels like too much *in* our bodies (grief, rage, anxiety) negative body image offers us a new pathway, something we can change *about* our bodies.

- **How does negative body image offer a form of hope?** When we believe that changing our bodies will change how we feel and how people respond to us, it gives us hope. We may not have control over our circumstances, but we can believe we can have control over our body. Focusing on our bodies offers hope that a future version of ourselves will have more of what we want. The problem is that future versions of ourselves are not in the present moment, with our present body and feelings. When we focus on our future body, our current emotional experiences don't get tended to.

To interrupt this cycle, we need to learn to honor what our body is holding and understand why hating it has felt helpful. Our mind may say our body is "wrong," "disgusting," "too big," or "too small," and we can learn to decode that into "sad," "lonely," "angry" or "scared." In this chapter, we will explain:

- How experiences in childhood and family dynamics can impact how we see and feel in our body.
- How experiences and emotions can get stuck *in* our bodies yet are expressed through our perceptions *of* our bodies.
- How, at any age, negative body image can try to step in to capture our focus when we feel overwhelmed and/or have a lack of support.
- How self-hate can offer a temporary sense of distraction and hope when we are faced with painful circumstances and experiences.
- How focusing on changing our bodies offers a way to manage challenges *in* our bodies such as illness or injury and transitions such as adolescence and aging.

Here is a vignette to demonstrate what we mean when we say that body image can be a *safe landing zone* for unprocessed emotions.

The Wrong Shirt

Jocelyn described feeling anxious every time she left her parents' house after a visit. *"Whenever I leave, I feel agitated and squirmy, my clothes don't feel right on my body, nothing feels right. I feel like I have gained 20 lbs every time I leave, like I am squishing out of my clothes. Last night I kept thinking, 'I am in the wrong clothes, I am in the wrong shirt, I can't get comfortable.' I got home and was so fixated on buying a new shirt. I spent two hours searching online, not knowing why all of a sudden this shirt felt so important."*

BodySelf: Jocelyn, could you write down the words that stood out to you in what you just described?

Jocelyn: *Sure … that nothing felt right, something felt wrong, unsettled, heavy. I felt uncomfortable and squirmy, like I was squeezing out of my shirt. What the heck?*

BodySelf: Could you take a minute and think about what the shirt search might have been trying to help with or fix?

Jocelyn: *It would be like pressing refresh on my computer. It would make the squirminess and the squeeziness go away. It would help me feel less uncomfortable, like something felt right, like something made sense.*

BodySelf: Great, so the new shirt would help with that heavy, squirmy, squeezy feeling? If the squirminess and squeeziness could talk, what would they say?

Jocelyn: *The squeeziness would say, "I don't want to live the way that my parents live. They are so stuck in their roles and rules and I feel so squeezed into their stagnant life when I am there." The squirminess would say "I want to make my own decisions, create my own rules. The way my parents live is so different from the way I want to live, and it makes me so uncomfortable to be there and see how unhappy they are, how little they want anything to change. I want to change and grow—that is why I feel so squirmy!"*

BodySelf: So how do you think the shirt shopping was trying to help?

Jocelyn: *It was reminding me that I have a choice. That I don't have to feel stuck, that I don't have to squeeze myself into a life that doesn't fit. I want to find ways to process how sad I am for them, but also trust that I am going to build a life that feels spacious and alive. It makes so much sense now that the shirts I was drawn to were loose fitting with vibrant patterns.*

It turns out that our body image thoughts have been telling a story that we haven't known how to listen to. We weren't taught to translate that "squeeziness" in our body might actually mean that we feel "squeezed" when we're in our parents' home. Feeling "squirmy" in our body is an appropriate response to feeling "squeezed into" a stagnant house. When we observe our body image with mindful awareness, curiosity and compassion, we can translate its messages and bring to life what our body has to tell us. Jocelyn's body image was trying to tell her that she was ready to start a new chapter, one that featured more flexibility and her body image was trying to get her there with a new shirt. Jocelyn realized that feeling stuffed into her shirt was code for, "I feel stuffed into my family's stuckness. I want something very different for myself, I want a bigger, bolder life—one that is the right size for me."

"Anything that stores information requires a physical record, whether that's zeros and ones on a microchip, hieroglyphics on a stone, ink on a page, or grooves on vinyl. Your implicit emotional memories have a physical record, too. They're stored in the neuromuscular patterns that affect virtually every tissue in your body."

Amanda Blake

How Storing Starts

Before we start learning to listen to our body image, it's important to understand why the body speaks in code in the first place. Emotional pain may start well before we are equipped to manage it. Consider your younger self, before you knew how to read or write, before you fully understood social conventions, before you went through those awful middle school years. At any of these points in childhood, you may have encountered strong feelings of disappointment, loss or anger. Maybe you experienced racism, sexism, homophobia or an illness. Maybe there was a divorce in your household, an abusive sibling, a struggle to excel in sports or in school, a bully or a shaming coach or teacher. Maybe your father was cold and distant. Maybe your mother could never be wrong or take responsibility for her hurtful actions. Maybe you had a brother or sister with a physical disability or emotional challenges who took most of the attention in the family.

These experiences are not uncommon, but these challenges are hard to know how to manage, especially when we are young. Children don't have the language or the emotional regulation skills to know how to navigate big feelings. Caregivers play a crucial role in helping us learn how to process and metabolize these emotions, letting us know that they really get what we are going through, helping us understand why we feel the way we do, and teaching us what to do about it. But what happens when the adults who are caring for us are not available and/or competent at navigating their own feelings, or are the source of our big emotions in the first place?

Caregivers don't have to be perfect by any means, but if they don't have the skills to manage their own emotions and if they are unpredictable and unreliable, we will likely seek alternative ways to protect and resource ourselves. What's so amazing about us when we're young is our natural instinct to adapt and to create a sense of safety. For many, focusing on our bodies offers a very accessible way to anchor ourselves. It can feel empowering to believe that changing our bodies can directly alleviate our hurt and suffering. It's compelling to imagine that if we fix or perfect our bodies, our primary relationships may change for the better and then we will feel more safety and acceptance. Pretty brilliant, right? And heartbreaking.

Let's consider a few reasons why, for children and youth, hating their body feels like an alluring answer for managing big feelings:

- As children, it can be terrifying to see our caregivers as deficient. It can give us a greater sense of control to see ourselves as the problem, our bodies as defective and imperfect, and changing them as a tool to manage our hurts and disappointments.

- When we grow up in an environment lacking a sense of safety, our body is an ever present companion. Turning to it again and again as a source of security and hope (if we fix it) offers us a reliable comfort.

- Our body can become a "feelings receptacle" when we haven't been invited or taught to process or express our emotions.

- Thinking about altering our body offers a hope that the feelings and pain that it is carrying might shift or disappear.

You may be wondering, is it always the parents or caregivers? And does it always begin at this early life stage? No, not always. There are many pathways to feeling stuck with big emotions, overwhelmed and unsure about how to find our way.

Consider how your unique family system and your caregivers navigated their emotions and did or didn't prepare you well for managing your own. This doesn't mean that parents need to be emotional experts or have been in therapy, but if they didn't have the capacity to metabolize their emotions in a healthy way and allow room for you to do the same, that can have a significant impact on you and how you navigate your feelings.

The BodySelf perspective is that caregivers do their best with what they have, and that their ancestors likely may have also faced unique challenges and had limited access to support. Our intention is never to blame, just to contextualize to generate a more accurate and compassionate narrative.

Exercise 4.1 Caregivers and Emotions

If it feels ok to you, try to remember how your primary caregivers managed their emotions.

How did they manage their sadness?

_____

_____

Their anger?

_____

_____

Their joy?

_____

_____

What did it feel like to be around them when they were having big feelings?

_____

_____

When you were upset as a child, how were your feelings of sadness, anger or overwhelm tended to?

_____

_____

Overall, what did you learn from your early caregivers about how to deal with your emotions?

_____

_____

What did you do when you had big feelings? Who did you turn to or how did you attempt to take care of those feelings?

_____

_____

What is it like to consider these things? We recognize that there are a range of ways these questions might make you feel. Taking a mindful moment to breathe, feel your feet on the floor, and place a hand on your heart or belly may be a compassionate way for you to close out this exercise.

Client Spotlight: Times Square Makes Me Feel Fat

Talia grew up feeling different from the rest of her family. Both of her parents and her older brother were intense, driven, and highly focused on status, achievement and self-improvement. Talia had a much softer presence and was drawn to quieter, more reflective activities and interactions. Because her family highly valued intellectual growth and professional achievement, her parents spent a lot of time and money keeping Talia busy with activities both after school and in the summer. This left Talia with little room for the quiet time her body and temperament longed for.

As Talia got older, she started to feel more critical of her body. For reasons she didn't understand at the time, she became fixated on her size. The more her family pushed her to be out in the world exploring and learning, the worse she felt about her body and the more she wanted to shrink.

Talia's family would go to New York City regularly, as they considered it a "cultural mecca" and her parents insisted that they stay right in the heart of the city in Times Square. In this environment, Talia was unbearably overstimulated, but there was no space in her family for those feelings. She felt like her body actually grew larger the closer they got to Manhattan. It felt like there was no room for her naturally slower rhythm and the energy of the city was filling her up like a balloon. Talia restricted her food intake whenever they were in NYC, because it felt like the only way to quiet how "fat" she felt. Years later, she was able to make the connection that her experiences of "feeling fat" growing up were much more about feeling "full" of stimulation and overwhelm than about her physical size.

"Locating the problem within the body simplifies for so many people what is wrong with their lives."

Jeanne Catanzaro

Our Ever-accessible Body

The body is one of our most accessible tools; it's local, it's here and now, and it's ours. By seeing our bodies as "imperfect," or "wrong," we have somewhere to focus our energy when strong feelings hit. Our bodies can feel like the paper on which we hope to rewrite our future. There are so many difficult experiences and seasons of our lives that might lead us to focus on our bodies, particularly given that we live in a culture where physical improvement is touted as the answer for almost everything. Our bodies are by, design, constantly changing, which makes them a perfect target for relentless self-improvement. The act of turning towards changing our bodies as a method for containing overwhelming feelings can happen at any stage of life.

Whether it's trying on a hundred different pairs of jeans, focusing on a new diet or just identifying parts of our bodies that need improvement, these are all ways that body image is trying to help us feel more or less of something. The formula is extraordinarily appealing in its simplicity. There are many life circumstances that might feel like too much and a body focus offers us a welcome distraction, even if it brings its own kind of suffering.

Client Spotlight: Everyone Knew How to Interact But Me

Ellie started experiencing depression and social anxiety when she was in the 7th grade. She felt "out of it," like all of her peers knew what was going on, but that she "didn't know how to be." She felt "weird and insecure," certain that people thought she was "stupid." At the same time, Ellie's parents were going through a contentious divorce and, so for Ellie, neither home nor school felt comfortable or reliable. Ellie's changing adolescent body felt like the only thing she had any control over and consequently, throughout high school, she calorie counted and body checked, trying to manage her body when nothing else made sense.

Ellie continued to struggle socially in college, and it wasn't until she entered a graduate program in clinical psychology that she was able to access psychological testing and discovered that she was on the autism spectrum. This information came as such a relief to Ellie; it gave language and a context for why she had struggled so much relationally and felt such social anxiety and depression early in her life. It also helped her understand why she had felt such a rigid attachment to her body size. She realized that focusing on her body had been an anchor when she had felt unmoored in her family and in her social life. Striving for an idealized body had offered her a way to feel like she could "fit in" and counterbalance her social disorientation and vulnerability. Over time, as she got more support through therapy and a group designed to teach relationship skills, she was able to soften her grip on her body size significantly.

Bodies and Underrepresentation

Many factors contribute to how we experience and view our bodies: societal culture, family culture, trauma, mental health challenges, physical disabilities, racism, sexism, homophobia, chronic illness, to name a few. Our unique body image story may feel especially vulnerable when we are part of an underrepresented group and don't look like the dominant culture. Sometimes, we decide that "fixing" the bodies that are the targets of judgment and discrimination might mute our pain and redirect our hurts and losses. The body can become the part of our life that we can change when the larger issues feel oppressive and out of our control.

- Lina had been working for years as a childcare worker, diligently following the protocols to attain her green card. It was a stressful and vulnerable process and along the way, she noticed how much more critical she had become of her body. As the process dragged on and she encountered more obstacles, focusing on her body felt like a path that had resolution in the midst of feeling stuck and hopeless about her citizenship.

- As a lesbian working in a primarily male construction company, Sam noticed how much her body image would change depending on the dynamics of her workday. When she was working on small independent projects, she felt strong and confident. On the days that she was at larger sites with an all-male team, many of whom would tease her, she found herself becoming self-critical. She started going to the gym every day after work, even when she was exhausted, with hopes that being in top physical form would somehow protect her from the hurtful jabs from her co-workers.

- As a single woman in her 40s who never wanted a husband or children, Michelle felt self-conscious that she was not on a traditional path and worried that people might wonder why. As a result, she worked hard to maintain a mainstream "ideal" physique and invested in a high-end wardrobe to offset some of the self-consciousness she felt about being different. It felt like a way she could show the world that she was relatable and "really had it together" even if she wanted an alternative lifestyle from that of her colleagues and friends.

- As a Black female executive in a white male-dominated corporation, Aaliyah felt a great deal of pressure to overperform. Although she was always well-prepared for meetings, she was routinely spoken over and given less consideration than her white, male colleagues. She poured her frustrated energy into her crossfit workouts where she was a leader and top performer. Aaliyah developed some significant injuries and noticed how reluctant she was to take time off because it felt so compelling to be seen and recognized for her skill and hard work at the gym.

Feeling unseen and misunderstood can leave us with a lot of painful feelings. Hyper focusing on our bodies can feel like a way to try to offset the pain that comes with the disparities we experience in our surroundings. Marginalization often leads to a sense of powerlessness. A body focus can offer us a sense of control.

Client Spotlight: Man Enough?

Alex had spent his early years feeling a great deal of conflict within his body, certain that living in the female body he was born into didn't feel right. Over time, it became clear that he felt most aligned with the male gender and changed his name, pronouns and wardrobe, but didn't feel drawn to change his body in any way. Living in an urban environment within a strong queer community, he felt comfortable in his body. He had made the changes that felt right to him.

Yet, when he returned to his parents' rural home to visit his more conservative family, he felt more vulnerable and body-conscious. He noticed that weeks before he was heading home for a holiday, he would become critical of his body and more ashamed that he didn't spend more time working out and bulking up. He felt a new urgency to look "more manly," though he wasn't sure why.

Over time, Alex realized that the pressure he felt to change his body before going home was linked to making his family more comfortable. He had grown up in an area where men typically looked a particular way and unconsciously had developed a belief that if he looked more traditionally male, his transition might make more sense to his family, particularly his three younger brothers. Alex hoped that if he came home with a more muscled physique, he would better fit in with his family.

Redirecting Our Pain

In addition to fantasizing about changing our body to redirect emotional upset, we may focus on body image to try to manage feelings related to health issues, injuries and chronic conditions. Channeling the grief, frustration and fear we feel *towards* our body's pain and/or limitations into something that feels more immediate and "resolvable" *about* our bodies can temporarily make those difficult emotions feel less overwhelming. For example:

- As a star on a Division 1 college basketball team, Ryall had a career ending knee injury that devastated him. He found himself obsessively researching fitness regimes and extreme diet plans. Thinking about making sure his body still looked "like a top athlete" offered a distraction from the grief of this major loss.

- Sarah had navigated Crohn's disease for most of her life and longed for a tiny waist, which, to her, symbolized freedom from the symptoms of bloating and abdominal discomfort she managed daily.

- Molly had suffered two miscarriages. When she was pregnant for the third time, she found herself ruminating nonstop about her weight. Was she gaining too much? Too little? Was she doing it "right?" It felt safer to direct her worry towards her body than address the deep fear she carried about losing another pregnancy.

Orienting ourselves during times of suffering through body control is compelling and initially can feel empowering. And at the same time, doing so keeps us from finding the support and resources we need to fully address and grieve what we are navigating.

Client Spotlight: North Star Stomach

Ariel had always wanted children from the time she was young. When she was a teen, she started to experience pain and discomfort during her menstrual cycle, which kept her in bed for multiple days each month. As she got older, the pain got worse and ultimately she was diagnosed with endometriosis. Doctors told her there was a strong likelihood that she would be unable to bear her own children. She began a journey of managing the disease with various treatments, procedures and surgeries which helped, but they did not give her the kind of pain relief she longed for. Among her symptoms was a great deal of pelvic pain, and she found herself becoming increasingly focused on having a "flat stomach." She had always felt self-conscious about her hips and belly and over time, achieving a flatter stomach became a sort of "North Star," a way to direct all the other feelings about her condition that were overwhelming. For Ariel, it felt like the goal of changing her stomach offered a way to manage the parts of her body that had brought her so much discomfort and loss.

"She's the only person I'll know my entire life and yet I sometimes talk to her like a useless appliance that doesn't work."

Mari Andrew

The Hope in Self-hate

Focusing on our body can help us manage a world that often feels unmanageable. Turning towards our imperfect bodies can feel like a "life raft" when things feel like too much. A part of us believes that if we change the outside, maybe something on the inside will feel different. If we are in the right body, it mitigates some other dynamic, worry or fear that we are carrying. This lines up perfectly with the cultural message that we need to close the gap between what we look like and the ideal, sparking hope for a better day by fixing and conforming. This strategy is particularly tempting and compelling if we were never taught how to manage our feelings, how to be seen or take up space, or how to skillfully resource ourselves.

Feeling unsatisfied when we examine the topography of our lives often leads us to feel unsatisfied with the topography of our bodies. Why? Because body hatred feels familiar and redirecting our hurts and relational losses towards our bodies gives us a sense of control and mastery. We can't tell you how many times we have heard some version of, "I feel so full! I know I have gained weight, my clothes are definitely tighter," in response to an overwhelming emotional experience. Feeling "full" of self-judgment is familiar, and offers the possibility of change, while feeling "full" of other emotions can just feel bad.

Client Spotlight: The Puffiness is the Pain

Dan was getting ready for dinner with his hypercritical father, who he saw only once a year when his dad was in town for a conference. Dan was dreading the evening. Dan found being around his dad painful and always left these dinners feeling defeated. His dad was a well-known surgeon who had always wanted Dan to follow in his footsteps and when Dan chose nursing, his father had openly expressed his disappointment. His father had acted as if his primary role as a parent was to ensure his son's success by pointing out the ways Dan needed to improve himself—in school, in sports, at work and his body. Dan's father would often make references to Dan "looking puffy" to express concerns about Dan's weight.

Dan had been working double shifts for the few weeks leading up to his dad's visit. He hadn't had any time for exercise or to prepare satisfying meals, so he had been eating at the hospital cafeteria or from vending machines. He had been tired and frustrated about his relentless work schedule, though it was only in the days leading up to seeing his father that the familiar self-hating language started to swirl in his head. Dan started feeling increasingly judgmental of himself and particularly his body. He was especially focused on how "puffy" he felt, even in his loose-fitting scrubs. He started to contemplate various ways that he could manage his body differently—getting up at 4 am to exercise or skipping meals—old strategies that he had left behind years ago. Dan's self-criticism tried to beat his father to the punch.

When Focusing on the Fix is the Fix

Criticizing our bodies and imagining ways to change them can also be an attempt to discharge the physical energy that accompanies our emotions. Focusing on the body is actually quite intuitive—a hug, a cry, a walk or belting out a song are healthy ways to utilize the body to discharge emotions. However, most of us weren't taught or coached in how to appropriately process our feelings so "fixing" our body can seem like a handy alternative. When we attempt to express, release and metabolize our suffering through changing our bodies—focusing on the fix is the fix.

Here's an outline of how this often plays out:

1 We have an experience that leaves us with BIG emotions.

2 We are not able to process our feelings and/or express them and we don't know how to resource ourselves.

3 Our body image steps in and we experience a BBIM: we redirect the emotion and energy of what we are feeling towards changing our bodies in an attempt to soothe, quiet, resolve or release what is happening emotionally.

For example, it might be easier to focus on the way we will look at our upcoming family reunion than to sit in the feelings of fear about messy family dynamics. We all know how good it feels to focus on an attainable task, particularly when other aspects of our lives feel "chaotic" or "out of control." Rerouting these physical sensations of overwhelm to "right" what feels "wrong" sidesteps the intense feelings and directs energy towards a more controllable and hopeful outcome.

Client Spotlight: Trying to Climb Out of the Pain

Martina grew up with a single father who was well-intentioned, but also poorly equipped for parenthood. Her mother passed away when she was ten, and her father had little skill or resources to help Martina through her grieving process. Martina felt disconnected in a household where no one spoke about things directly and although she didn't have words to explain it at the time, she knew something inside her felt intolerable. She discovered rock climbing at the local gym in high school and it was a welcome outlet. Climbing was a great resource for Martina, it offered her a sense of control and a way to feel grounded when home felt so unwelcoming. But over time, climbing became her primary focus, and while it felt compelling, Martina was far less connected to her friends and other aspects of her life.

Martina joined a grief group in college and with this support, she learned to put words to her experience growing up. "When I was a teenager, I had all this grief, anger and sadness, but I didn't know what to do with these feelings. There was nobody to talk to about it or even notice what was happening. Exercise was the only way I knew to get the icky feelings out of me. But each morning, I would wake up with the feelings all over again. When I didn't train, I felt uncomfortably full and so critical of that feeling."

Martina sought out a therapist who specialized in mindfulness and emotional regulation. Over time, she gained new skills for recognizing and managing her emotions. "Now when I visit with my dad, I feel deeply uncomfortable, agitated and grumpy and I just want the visit to be over. For years sitting with him made me feel "fat". Now I can see how lonely I felt growing up, how much I longed for him to see me and that I had no way to express what I was feeling inside. I know now that being around him was really painful and it left me full of emotions and climbing was the only way I knew to manage them.

"Now, even though I feel agitated and sad when I am around him, I know it is progress to sense what is actually going on inside me and to know when I leave, that it is crucial to find ways to take good care of my agitated and grumpy self."

Exercise 4.2 BodySelf Mad Libs

For each person the motives behind the desired "fix" can be different, though the intention remains consistent. In order to get more clear on our patterns, try this exercise.

If my _____ [body or body part] is _____ [adjective], I will feel more _____ [adjective].

Example:

"If my butt is smaller and less squishy, I will feel more elegant and powerful."

Try it again with a different body part:

If my _____ [body or body part] is _____ [adjective], I will feel less _____ [adjective].

Example:

"If my belly is less flabby, I will feel less old and invisible."

A focus on our body offers a simple, immediate, and clear solution. It offers temporary relief from our overwhelming emotions by focusing on something else and the hope that once we fix our body, things will feel different. The problem is that this plan often takes us on endless loops and doesn't allow us the time or space to process, solve, or heal whatever is driving the desire to change our body.

We hope it is starting to make sense why a focus on hating our body, seeing ourselves as flawed and trying to improve ourselves might feel compelling and adaptive. We feel pain and we try to manage it by focusing on what we can change about ourselves, and as an added bonus, society claps. However, this strategy doesn't make the problem go away. In fact, it prevents us from attending to the emotional impact of the problem. The real issue never gets our presence, our attention or our compassion. Heroically, our body image offered itself up to give us a sense of hope and a way to feel distracted and held in a painful yet very familiar pattern. Let's map your unique body image cycle and see how this plays out for you.

We like to use the metaphor of a rotary to explain why these patterns are so compelling and how easily we can get caught up in a "fix it" mindset about our bodies. When in our day to day travels we hit "bumps," aka experiences that are painful, hurtful or overwhelming, we divert from the present moment to avoid what we are feeling and unknowingly enter the body image rotary. Rotaries are circular intersections, offering multiple "entrances" and "exits," and the potential to loop round and round endlessly. Once we enter a rotary, these "fix-it choices" are compelling and distract us from the uncomfortable experience that prompted us to take the rotary exit in the first place.

The Typical Rotary Cycle

- You experience overwhelming feelings in response to something in your life.
- Your big feelings, thoughts and sensations get redirected towards your body, aka a BBIM.
- You decide to fix your body and create a plan.
- You get focused on the action (diet, exercise, etc) and distracted from the overwhelming feelings.
- The emotions that are fueling bad body image don't get addressed.
- A pattern for fixing the body in response to uncomfortable feelings gets laid down and is likely to repeat.
- Broader culture is likely to reinforce fixing the body as "healthy."

The Negative Body Image Rotary

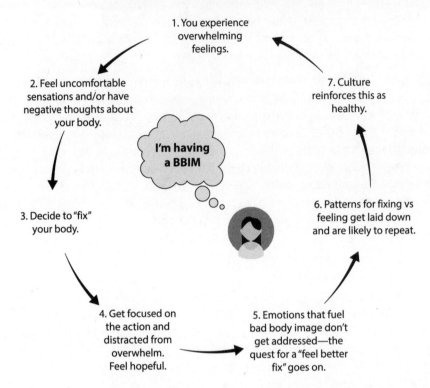

1. You experience overwhelming feelings.

2. Feel uncomfortable sensations and/or have negative thoughts about your body.

7. Culture reinforces this as healthy.

I'm having a BBIM

3. Decide to "fix" your body.

6. Patterns for fixing vs feeling get laid down and are likely to repeat.

4. Get focused on the action and distracted from overwhelm. Feel hopeful.

5. Emotions that fuel bad body image don't get addressed—the quest for a "feel better fix" goes on.

It makes a lot of sense that we may want to reroute or take a different path when things feel like too much. So many options, so many ways to think about changing ourselves! Of course, if we stay on this rotary for too long, we never get the opportunity to 1) understand what is driving the "fix it" quest 2) learn to process our emotions or 3) tend to problems that diverted us to the rotary in the first place.

The rotary exercise below serves as the foundation of all our workshops, it allows us to map out the way that critical thoughts about our body may reroute our thinking to protect us from our pain. Breaking down our "body image rotaries" can offer insight into how our negative body image thoughts have been trying to help us navigate more than we realize.

Exercise 4.3 What Does this Body Image Rotary Look Like for You?

Pick a recent BBIM.

Describe it:

_____

_____

You experience overwhelming feelings. You find yourself in a BBIM. How do you know you are in a BBIM? What are you thinking or feeling?

_____

_____

You experience negative sensations and/or thoughts about your body. Your negative thoughts or sensations are:

_____

_____

You decide to fix your body and create a plan. Your go-to fix-it plan is:

_____

_____

You feel hopeful things will feel different. What are you hoping for?

_____

_____

Are there places or people that reinforce these choices as "healthy" or good?

_____

_____

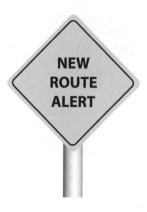

How to BodySelf your Rotary

Here is what it looks like to bring the BodySelf approach to your Rotary experience:

- You experience overwhelming feelings.
- Your big feelings, thoughts, and sensations get redirected towards your body, aka a BBIM.
- You decide to fix your body and create a plan.
- ~~You get focused on the action (diet, exercise, etc) and distracted from the overwhelming feelings.~~
- ~~The emotions that are fueling bad body image don't get addressed and continue to drive a body fix.~~
- ~~A pattern for fixing the body gets laid down and is likely to repeat.~~
- ~~Broader culture is likely to reinforce fixing the body as "healthy."~~
- Now let's bring in the BodySelf approach: Use *mindful awareness* to recognize you are in a pattern.
- *Get curious*. Ask yourself, what might be *triggering* me? Why is my *body image so loud* right now?
- *Bring compassion*. Recognize that these patterns are driven by emotional pain and you have the ability to support yourself.

The BodySelf Rotary

1. You experience overwhelming feelings.

2. Feel uncomfortable sensations and/or have negative thoughts about your body.

I'm having a BBIM

6. Ask judgment to step aside. **Offer compassion**.

3. Decide to "fix" your body.

5. **Get curious**. What else might be going on? Why is body image loud right now?

4. Recognize you are in an old pattern and remember you can BodySelf this moment.

CHANGE AHEAD

Exercise 4.4 BodySelf Your Rotary Cycle: Part 1

- You experience overwhelming feelings.
- Your big feelings, thoughts and sensations get redirected towards your body, aka a BBIM.
- You decide to fix your body and create a plan.
- ~~You get focused on the action (diet, exercise, etc) and distracted from the overwhelming feelings.~~
- ~~The emotions that are fueling bad body image don't get addressed and continue to drive a body fix.~~
- ~~A pattern for fixing the body gets laid down and is likely to repeat.~~
- ~~Broader culture is likely to reinforce fixing the body as "healthy."~~

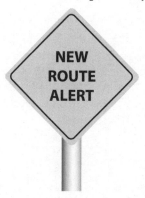

*Start with **mindful awareness**: You recognize you're in your Rotary. You decide not to continue and you pause. You observe how you are thinking about your body and notice what sensations you are experiencing.*

_____

_____

Example:

"I just put in an offer to buy my first home. I feel incredibly excited and at the same time, terrified. I find myself thinking a lot about my stomach and how big it feels, really focusing on how much bigger it looks."

Get curious: *Ask yourself, what might be triggering me? Why is my body image so loud right now? What is going on in this moment that might be leading me towards a body image focus?*

_____

_____

Example:

"After years of saving, searching and deliberating, I just put an offer to buy my first home. It feels incredibly exciting and at the same time terrifying. Is this the right decision? All I want to think about is fixing my stomach."

Offer compassion. *Invite a compassionate lens to your Rotary and ask any judgment to step aside. How might compassion respond to you and where you have landed on your rotary?*

_____

_____

Example:

"It makes so much sense that I am freaking out. This is the biggest decision I have ever made alone. Focusing on my stomach is an old habit that feels compelling in its simplicity right now when there is so much in my life that feels new and unknown."

This is not the last you will see of your rotary. We are going to continue to teach you skills to deepen your ability to take good care of the needs and wants your body image has tried so hard to help with.

*Bless all that your body holds: the history,
the present, the undiscovered.*

*May you recognize in the coming days and weeks when
your negative body image cycles intervene to help you.*

*May the well-worn paths of body hatred yield
to new discoveries and clarity.*

*Bless you with courage and softness, as you step out
of habit and into something unknown, yet decidedly
in the direction of YOU.*

5 | Body Image and Relationships
Mirroring and Shapeshifting

"Know that the desire to be perfect is probably the veiled expression of another desire—to be loved."

Ron Padgett, "How to Be Perfect", from *Collected Poems*
(Coffee House Press, 2013)

Body Image and Relationships

What about body image *isn't* about relationships? Our body image can be profoundly impacted by how accurately we are seen by the people closest to us, whether we feel a sense of belonging, whether we have permission to feel our feelings and what kind of relationship we have with ourselves. In this chapter we will explore how:

- "Mirroring" is something that starts happening early on with our caregivers, before we ever even knew how to admire or criticize our bodies.
- "Shapeshifting" can be an early strategy to try to protect ourselves or preserve our relationships within our family and over time, shapeshifting can impact how we see and/or feel about our bodies.
- We often "cut and paste" our early emotional shapeshifting patterns onto our adult relationships.
- There is an important interplay between our relationships and how we see and think about our bodies. As adults, we have choices about which "relational mirrors" support our BodySelf.

Mirroring

As babies, our earliest mirrors didn't have reflective glass or gold frames. They were our caregivers. Long before we started the endless two-step in front of a physical mirror—deciding whether we looked fat or thin, pretty or ugly—our caregivers were reflecting our image back at us. Through their expressions, actions and reactions, our caregivers gave us a way to interpret who we were and what we were capable of—no matter how well they were up to the task. Some of them were distracted, defended, or dealing with their own traumas, addictions, or illnesses, and therefore could not "mirror" us well. As a result, we might have gotten the message that our needs, joys, fears and sorrows were invisible to them, or just didn't matter. Somehow we had to figure out how to get our needs met and tend to our loneliness; the accessibility and proximity of our body made it a natural place to turn.

"In individual emotional development, the precursor of the mirror is the mother's (caregiver's) face."

D. W. Winnicott

Instinctively, children's primary orientation is to be safe. Far before we understand intellectually what is going on, we attune to what is happening around us. We sense dynamics within the family that are askew and/or relationships that are in conflict. To increase stability in our family, we may adapt by "reshaping" ourselves based on what is needed using our own natural skill sets. Because as children we don't have a lot of relational tools at our disposal, we aim to improve family dynamics with a simple strategy: changing the "shape" of *how* we show up in our family system.

Shapeshifting

You may have heard the term "shapeshifting" in the context of mythology, folklore or even superheroes. A person or animal attempts to address a challenge in their storyline by taking on a new form, one better suited for the dilemma at hand. Similarly, we "reshape ourselves" to improve the dynamics in our early relationships. "Shapeshifting" often develops long before we understand what is happening or why we are doing it. Shapeshifting our behavior, thoughts and values can be a way to respond to and navigate through our early relationships when things feel unsafe or disconnected. Shapeshifting takes many forms: shrinking our needs, silencing ourselves, expanding our success or cultivating a skill like caretaking. While the shapes may be different, the transformations are in service of accessing more connection with an individual family member or creating more stability within the family as a whole.

- Danny was a sensitive child with a fierce talent for humor. When his mom's anxiety threatened to shut down her ability to function, he could sense it and rushed in to entertain her. Sometimes this was enough to bring her mood up and refocus her. He would step into "showtime" mode whenever he sensed she needed it, even if that was not what he wanted to do.

- Isla grew up with a mother who worked as a social worker in the foster care system. Often, her mom would take Isla's clothing and toys and give them to her young clients, saying it was the right thing to do because Isla had so much more than they did. Isla became confused about her own desires for the new things her friends had, wondering if she was greedy and selfish. She stopped asking for anything new from her mother and instead took her friends' hand-me-downs.

- Jonathan grew up with a single mom who raised him and his two siblings. With her demanding corporate job and late hours, his mom rarely made it to her kids' games and extracurricular performances. Jonathan and his siblings each got to pick one event a quarter that she would come to. When Jonathan's mom didn't make it to his play because of a last minute board meeting, he told her how sad this made him. Watching her tired eyes tear up that night, he vowed never to share his disappointment with her again.

Shapeshifting initially plays out emotionally as we try to adapt to the dynamics around us. Let's explore how you may have shapeshifted in your early years to adapt to your environment.

Exercise 5.1 Shapeshifting Check-in

The following questions invite you to learn more about your early shapeshfiting patterns.

Growing up, did you sense that there were relational imbalances and or conflicts in your family? If so, how did that affect you?

_____

_____

Were there relationships for which you altered your emotional "shape"—needs, boundaries, expressions or expectations? Which ones?

_____

_____

How did you change the shape of your expectations, boundaries, needs?

_____

_____

What do you think your shapeshifting was trying to get you? Approval, love, connection or something else?

_____

_____

Puzzle Piecing

We like to use the metaphor of a puzzle to capture the ways we may shapeshift to try to preserve a relationship and/or try to protect our family as a whole in some way. Think of each family as a puzzle and each family member, including yourself, as a piece within that puzzle.

Two Puzzle Pieces (One Relationship)

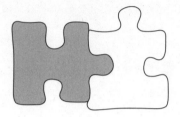

One shapeshifting pattern is contorting our feelings, needs and gifts in a specific relationship within our family to attempt to fit into/connect with the larger puzzle. This might look like:

- Keeping our feelings, needs or opinions to ourselves because a family member responds negatively to them.
- Over-indexing a talent or trait because it is positively received and rewarded.
- Spending much of our energy attuning to a family member to anticipate and attend to their unpredictable mood.
- Diminishing our needs to make room for a family member's physical or mental illness.
- A combination of some or all of these strategies.

Remember, as children, much of the information we took in was through the sensations of our body. We didn't track everything in the form of concrete memories. While this list represents common strategies, there are many ways a younger authentic self can change the shape of their needs, longings and behaviors to attempt to stay connected with a family member.

Client Spotlight: Basement Bonding

José longed to be closer to his older brother, Luis. Their father was in the military; he was often deployed, and when he was home, was exhausted and distracted. Their mom was warm and charming with others when they were at church or social events in the community, but she was self-involved and unavailable at home. This left José feeling alone, like no one was tracking him or curious about who he was or what he was interested in.

Of all his family members, José felt his older brother, Luis, was his best hope for a caring relationship. Luis, was a charismatic guy who really loved José and lived at home and attended a local community college to save money. Whenever Luis was home, he was usually in the family's basement with his friends, watching sports, playing video games and sometimes drinking. José started joining them, often choosing basement hang-out time over homework. He pretended to be interested and engaged in whatever Luis and his friends were doing, even though he didn't love sports, had only a vague interest in video games, and usually felt more tired than buzzed from beer. José was interested in science and wanted to be a marine biologist but kept all of that to himself. When his grades started to slide, he was referred to a school counselor who helped José understand what was hard for him at home. The counselor also connected José with a school club with kids who shared his interests, as well as a volunteer job at the local aquarium. José started to build his own identity and connections and while he still wanted a close relationship with his brother, he was no longer trying to shapeshift himself to get it.

"Pain travels through families until someone is ready to feel it."

Stephi Wagner, Founder – Mother Wound Project

The Family Puzzle

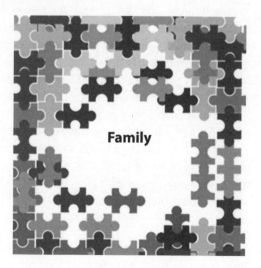

Family

Every family is a puzzle. Shapeshifting can also play out by changing our puzzle piece to impact our family "puzzle" as a whole. We may come to believe that by changing the shape of our individual puzzle piece, we can address and even resolve the issues, imbalances and deficiencies within the larger "puzzle." This adaptation is a way to feel control over what is challenging in the larger dynamic.

Here are a few examples:

- Overachieving in academics, athletics or some other arena because the family values it.
- Shrinking back so as not to get any negative attention.
- Becoming overly responsible for household duties, organization and overall functionality of the home.
- Silencing feelings, needs, and longings because caregivers have limited capacity to see and respond to them.
- Contributing to a family value of financial or social status.
- Investing energy in mediating or peacekeeping between caregivers and/or siblings.
- Compensating for a sibling who is struggling with physical or mental health challenges by being "easy."
- Going along with family traditions or behaviors even if it feels dramatically misaligned, unenjoyable or uncomfortable.

Client Spotlight: Filling the Space Between Them

From a young age, Bella was aware that she could "light her parents up." They called their only child "Superstar." Her mom battled depression for most of her adult life and over time, her dad became less and less engaged with the family. Both of her parents were unhappy, and Bella found herself feeling more and more compelled not only to cheer them up but to try to bring them back together. She knew how much her mom longed for her dad to be more attentive. She saw how powerless her dad felt when her mom was in a period of depression. Bella felt the energy in the room change when she walked in; her mom livened up and her dad softened. While this felt good in the moment, over time it left her feeling an increasing level of responsibility. It seemed like there was a gaping hole between her parents and her dynamism was the only thing that could fill it. Her natural affinity for humor and charm felt like it had morphed into one big performance. What once felt like a joyful aspect of her personality had grown into a family obligation.

There are many ways that we may shapeshift ourselves to stay connected with our families. Although these strategies may temporarily improve an individual or family relationship, they can't change the other person or family system and often become established relational patterns inside of us.

Exercise 5.2 Puzzle Piecing Mad Libs

We want to invite you to get curious about how early dynamics impacted the shape of your puzzle piece. This could be with:

- One particular family member (two puzzle pieces)
- Between you and your family dynamics as a whole (the family puzzle).

Two puzzle pieces

In my family I often shapeshifted my puzzle piece to better connect with

_____

To connect to the puzzle piece of _____ *I would*

_____

What I hoped to gain by shapeshifting was:

_____

The impact of my shapeshifting on the relationship was:

_____

The impact of shapeshifting on me was:

_____

Looking back, when I shapeshifted I ended up:

_____

Example:

In my family I often shapeshifted my puzzle piece to better connect with: my mom.

To connect to the puzzle piece of my mom *I would:* be quiet and agreeable.

What I hoped to gain by shapeshifting was: to prevent blow-ups.

The impact of my shapeshifting on the relationship was: that I shut down around her.

The impact of shapeshifting on me was: that I rarely expressed how I felt around people like her.

Looking back, when I shapeshifted I ended up: creating a belief that I should always become quiet and keep my opinions to myself when I'm around anyone who is explosive.

The family puzzle

I would use these three adjectives to describe my family puzzle

1. _____ 2. _____ 3. _____

I changed my puzzle piece to try to positively impact the family system as a whole by: _____

_____

Changing myself in this way impacted me in the following ways:

_____

What I really most wanted from the puzzle I was born into was:

_____

The following triggers are most likely to prompt me to return to my early puzzle piece shape:

_____

Example:

I would use these three adjectives to describe my family puzzle:

1. under-resourced   2. huge   3. chaotic

I changed my puzzle piece to try to positively impact the family system as a whole by:

caretaking and being "easy."

Changing myself in this way impacted me in that:

I would automatically go into people-pleasing mode and wasn't very connected to what I wanted.

What I most wanted from the puzzle I was born into was:

for them to value and know me outside of my caretaker role.

The following triggers are most likely to prompt me to return to my early puzzle piece shape:

chaotic bosses who value my ability to perform well without much support or training.

"Our bodies take on the shape of our repeated emotional experiences."

Amanda Blake

Embodying the Puzzle Piece

Regularly changing the size of our needs, longings and desires can easily evolve into shapeshifting the size and form of our physical bodies. Our emotional attempts at shapeshifting can't resolve the relational issues we face, so we may turn to what is accessible and in our control. Cultural messages hand us a shapeshifting map from a young age, reiterating the idea that changing our shape will change our lives for the better. Whether it is by shrinking, growing or perfecting, shapeshifting can be a strategy to manage *inside us* what feels intolerable *around us*. Changing our shape can give us hope for changing our relationships.

Client Spotlight: In the Long Run

Ryan ran cross-country for his high school team. Because he didn't excel at traditional sports in grade school, he was surprised to find he was particularly well-suited for cross country. Ryan loved being outside, being part of a team and the routine of daily practice. Increasingly, he was fed by the identity of being a good athlete. Having grown up with an older sister with a chronic illness that took much of his parents' time and attention, he loved all the visibility he got when he medaled at an event. He enjoyed being the one to set the pace for practices and was one of the best performers on the team. Though humble in nature, he relished the praise and attention he received as a celebrated athlete.

When his progress plateaued, as is typical for endurance athletes, he desperately searched for a way to get faster. He focused on getting leaner to try to pick up some speed. While he found himself distracted and irritable, focusing on his weight did give him a temporary hope that he could improve even more. A few weeks later, he got injured and couldn't run for the rest of the season.

The loss of his sport identity hit him hard, and he felt invisible again. Ryan was crushed and opened up to one of his teachers who encouraged him to talk to a school counselor. Through their conversations, Ryan was able to see the ways he benefited from his cross-country team experience, and the ways his star status had given him the attention and celebration he couldn't get given the burdens his family was dealing with.

Exercise 5.3 Embodied Puzzle Piece Mad Libs

We invite you to get curious about how your early shapeshifting patterns may have impacted your body image. Again, this embodied shapeshifting pattern may play out with an individual family member or the family system as a whole.

Embodied puzzle piece (one relationship)

My focus on my body image helped me better deal with my relationship with:

_____

My body image focus was trying to help me by:

_____

What I hoped to gain by shapeshifting my body was:

_____

Looking back, when I shapeshifted I ended up:

_____

Example:

My focus on my body image helped me better deal with my relationship with:
my dad.
My body image focus was trying to help me by:
showing him how disciplined, in control and driven I was.
What I hoped to gain by shapeshifting was:
his approval.
Looking back, when I shapeshifted, I ended up:
feeling like my body needed "fixing" and disconnecting from how I really felt.

Family-embodied puzzle piece

My focus on my body image helped me better deal with my family by:

_____

My body image focus was trying to help me by:

_____

What I hoped to gain by shapeshifting my body was:

_____

What I most wanted to avoid was:

_____

What I really wanted most from the puzzle I was born into was:

_____

Looking back, when I shapeshifted I ended up:

_____

Example:

My focus on my body image helped me better deal with my relationship with my family by:

giving me a day to day focus and hope that I could feel more appreciated.

My body image focus was trying to help me:

by giving me something to turn to when I felt lost and alone.

What I hoped to gain by shapeshifting my body was:

to be appreciated and adored.

What I most wanted to avoid was:

feeling lonely and unseen/unappreciated.

What I really wanted most from the puzzle I was born into was:

to be appreciated, supported and connected with.

Shapeshifting Over Time

The habit of changing ourselves and our body to improve our relationships can morph into a relational pattern that repeats throughout our lives. While we may have developed these formulas in our family of origin, they will likely stick with us as we grow older and be applied to other relational dynamics at work, with friends and romantic partners. We can start to navigate life with a belief that there is a correlation between our body and what happens in our relationships; that body shapeshifting is a dial we (often unconsciously) use to influence relational outcomes. Our shapeshifting parts may still be working hard to protect our younger selves, not having gotten the memo that we have aged and become more resourceful. This explains why what may feel like a minor issue with a friend or colleague can elicit a BBIM! Our current relationships may echo the ones that we shapeshifted for growing up, triggering our negative body image to spring into action. When this happens ... wham, bam, BBIM!

Client Spotlight: Bodies and Boundaries

Jasmine's parents divorced when she was a toddler, and she was primarily raised by her father. Her dad tried hard to show up for Jasmine and her younger brother and hide his depression, but he was always changing jobs and they moved frequently. Jasmine loved to dance and wherever they moved, she joined the dance club at the school or found a local class. It felt like her one anchor when so much around her was always changing. In high school, it felt harder to leave friends and more anxiety-provoking to make new ones. She found herself increasingly driven to achieve a "dancer's body," chasing a lean and muscular frame. It was a welcome focus amidst the chaos of her family life and felt like an investment in her identity as a dancer.

She received a scholarship to a college in a small town, and this finally gave her more stability. As she settled into a more predictable life, she recognized how her body focus had served her all those years. She felt much less compelled to perfect her body and enjoyed the creativity and camaraderie of dance.

In her senior year, she moved into a new apartment with two roommates who had already been living together. Oddly, the room she moved into didn't have a door. Initially, she was concerned, but the prior roommate had used a curtain and it seemed worth trying, given that it had been so hard to find an apartment she liked at a price she could afford. Pretty quickly though, Jasmine found herself feeling unwelcome and excluded by her roommates. They spoke in hushed tones around her and when they did engage with her, it was usually some sort of criticism. When they complained that her music was too loud, she reiterated her desire for a door and asked if the building manager had responded to their multiple emails. Jasmine tried to problem solve, but neither roommate was willing to contribute time or money to resolving the situation.

Over the course of the next few months, this feeling of being unwelcome intensified. For the first time in years, she found herself focusing on her weight, fantasizing about dieting and joining a gym in addition to her beloved dance classes. Jasmine reached back to these old shapeshifting strategies to try to manage the painful dynamics in her apartment. It wasn't until she moved out that she was able to see that her body focused shapeshifting strategies were trying to give her a sense of stability.

When Body Image Speaks in Relationships

When we habitually shapeshift, we inadvertently and unconsciously train ourselves to hide or override our truth. Yet our truth always lives in us and without a direct outlet, it may try to communicate through our body image. In uncomfortable or misaligned relational situations, body image generously offers to reroute our truth into body criticism. These signals may show up in situations where it is not safe or encouraged to be honest, or where our needs aren't acknowledged or attended to. This could be due to family, workplace, gender, race or relational dynamics, where there are negative consequences if we speak up for ourselves or violate unspoken rules and expectations. "I hate the way I look" may be the acceptable and habitual translation of "I hate the way you make me feel." When we are with someone who doesn't allow room for our experience or opinion, our body will communicate its discomfort to us. We may call this feeling "stuffed," "squishy" or "gross." Our body is telling us something isn't right. *The trick is to not mistake this for being something not right about us.*

Client Spotlight: No Space for Me

Jess's mom was highly anxious and overwhelmed and from a young age, Jess took on the role of both mother's helper and therapist. Not only did she help her mom manage the household, but Jess felt responsible for managing her mom's anxiety. Jess felt "weighed down and full" after these ongoing support sessions and she spent much of her childhood and adolescence feeling self-conscious about her body.

Jess was thrilled when she secured a job in San Francisco soon after graduating from college. She loved exploring this colorful new city, had made new friends quickly, and noticed how much more accepting she felt towards her body in her expansive new life.

When Jess's mom came to visit, she insisted on staying in Jess's studio apartment. Within minutes of her mom's arrival, her mom's anxiety filled the small space. It felt to Jess like the walls were closing in on her and there was no room left for her or the new life she was building. This frustrated, trapped feeling was all too familiar. Quickly, Jess's critical body monologue reappeared, and stayed loud through the weekend and even a few days beyond her mother's visit.

Jess had recently started with a new counselor through work and together they identified Jess's longtime role as her mom's mental health sherpa, carrying the feelings her mom could not and then redirecting her anger about it towards herself. It hadn't been safe or effective to share them in her family system—if Jess said anything honest, she would end up having to mop up her mom's feelings again. For Jess, rerouting all of her unexpressed emotions into negative thoughts about her body had been highly adaptive growing up. Feeling trapped in the small studio with her mother's abundant anxiety and unmet needs was deeply uncomfortable for Jess and it was also profoundly illuminating—it helped her understand how much her negative body image had been trying to help her all those years.

It is a BodySelf triumph to leave an uncomfortable encounter feeling attuned to our genuine experience. Naming, "I feel so angry that they kept talking over me and didn't ask a thing about me. I feel frustrated and kinda slimy," is progress! It means we didn't convert our negative feelings into body criticism. We were able to accurately interpret what our body was saying *to us, not about us*. This shift takes practice and the best place to start is to notice your relationship-inspired BBIMs: when they happen and to break them down with your BodySelf muscles: mindfulness awareness, curiosity and compassion. The more you can start to notice your physical sensations in these uncomfortable moments, the more you can notice what isn't feeling right. From there, with more clarity, you can figure out your next move, whether that be to speak up or find other ways to take care of yourself in response to the dynamic.

Exercise 5.4 BBIM = Shapeshifting Check-In

A relational conflict could be with anyone: a coach, a boss, an auto mechanic or even a professor. Even if it doesn't initially make sense to you why you may be experiencing vulnerability that leads to a Bad Body Image Moment, that's OK! Remember we are looking to surface the invisible pattens with our mindful awareness and our curiosity. It may be that your BBIM is in response to the feeling about the dynamic, not the person, so the next time you leave an interaction followed by a BBIM, ask yourself:

How did it feel to be with that person? Three adjectives:

1. _____ 2. _____ 3. _____

What sensations was I or am I feeling?

_____

_____

Did I get to show up in that interaction as myself?

_____

If not, what did I hold back?

_____

_____

What truth was not allowed to be said?

_____

_____

*What do I feel too **full** of (that isn't food)?*

_____

_____

*What do I need **more** of (that isn't food)?*

_____

_____

*When I sit with this person, what about them makes me uncomfortable and feels **misaligned**? (instead of thinking "what is misaligned about me or my body?")*

_____

_____

> *"Because true belonging only happens when we present our authentic, imperfect selves to the world, our sense of belonging can never be greater than our level of self-acceptance."*
>
> Brené Brown, Daring Greatly

Shapeshifting and Romance

In dating, and in many other relational dynamics, managing our bodies is an attempt to improve chances for acceptance and connection. It can feel empowering to think that by changing the shape of our bodies, we can manage the uncomfortable, magical and terrifying aspects of exploring new relationships. Why else would we spend endless hours trying to nail the perfect outfit and believe that if we didn't look right we might not get a second date?

Even if a new romantic relationship doesn't trigger familial wounds, we often engage in mental and physical gymnastics to appear like we have it "together." We try to be the breezy Instagram version of ourselves until the relationship develops more safety.

Client Spotlight: Out of Sync

Sam and David started dating soon before David moved to another state for graduate school. They really cared for one another and wanted to give a long distance relationship a try. Sam was a musician and had an unstructured schedule, often waking up late, eating only one or two big meals out and staying out late at night, either performing or practicing with his band. David, on the other hand, loved the structure of grad school and his daily routines. When David visited, Sam's routine was initially fun and exciting, but over time David started to notice how the differences in their lifestyles affected him. David could never quite shift sleep schedules so never got enough sleep, and he wasn't used to eating out and constantly being around people. After his visits with Sam, David was not only exhausted, he actually felt like his body was changing. He found himself much more body conscious and had thoughts that he should be working out more to compensate. Whenever he would spend a weekend synced up with Sam's life rhythm, David would leave feeling really badly about his body.

David was falling for Sam and didn't quite know how to share what he was experiencing. He was afraid of risking his connection with Sam or embarrassing himself by being "too sensitive." In trying to adapt to Sam's schedule, David was overriding his own body cues and needs and his body image was letting him know he was out of alignment. Ultimately, David shared his worries with Sam and they were able to negotiate the structure of their visits so they both felt like they got what they needed. Not surprisingly, as David opened up more to Sam about what he needed, his negative body image settled significantly.

The Double Whammy Factor: Size As Currency

Much in the same way that athletic, academic or financial success can be a strong family value, weight and/or size can also be a family standard by which one is "measured." An over-investment in size is often driven by a desire to feel accepted, valued and/or celebrated within the family. In fact, in some families, a specific size can be a family currency that trickles down through generations and impacts the family puzzle. We often meet clients who realize that an overinvestment in their size is driven by a desire to be celebrated and valued by their family. For example:

- Both of Mia's parents were exceptional runners who met at a track and field World Championship. Even though Mia was not a competitive athlete by nature, she felt pressure to be on the school track team and to have a lean body type like all the runners her parents hung out with. Secretly, however, she preferred slower-paced activities like walking and baking.

- Dina's parents divorced when she was five, leaving her mom to manage almost everything for her and her younger sisters. Her dad was uninvolved and spent most of his free time compulsively exercising and perfecting his body. Because he was so disengaged with his daughters in most aspects of their lives, the one place they subconsciously had hopes for creating more connection was through exercise. Dina and her sisters tried to make their bodies "fit" his ideal with hopes he would be more interested in them and their lives.

It's a double whammy when we are influenced both by the broader cultural ideals of what a body should look like, as well as the culture of our family. We find it valuable to get clear on which messages are coming from each culture. When body size or shape is a valuable currency in a family, it can lead to:

- Struggling to accept your body type if it is different from the family's ideal.

- Feeling like you're not fully accepted in your family if you don't fall within their body standards.

- Feeling like there is a family investment in your being a particular size which can come to feel like a responsibility or burden.

- Disliking certain body parts that either fit into your family ideal or are different.

- Assuming that these standards will determine your value and acceptance outside your family.

Client Spotlight: If You Fit in Then I am OK

Sonia's family immigrated to the U.S. when she was a child and it was a difficult transition, especially for her mom, Maria. Maria had lost her own mother at a young age and had been raised by various family members, often moving and changing schools. For Maria, moving to the U.S. felt like being displaced again, and it was overwhelming. She was deeply driven to make sure that Sonia fit in and never felt the way she had growing up. Maria associated living in the U.S. with a certain body type she had seen on TV growing up and made the assumption that the best way to ensure that Sonia transitioned well was to be in the "right clothes and the right body."

Sonia lived in the curvier body, which her mom associated with their native country and feared it might prevent Sonia from being accepted in her new peer group. Sonia's body was constantly under Maria's scrutiny, and because Sonia didn't understand what was driving her mom's intense investment in her body shape, she felt like she wasn't enough and that she needed to be vigilant about her weight to be loved by her mom and accepted by others.

Sometimes, a family value of a certain size or body type can be an attempt to address a parent's dissatisfaction with their own body. This is often connected to a parent's unaddressed trauma or other mental health issue. Parents and caregivers may have come to believe body perfection was the answer to their own suffering. If they don't address this within themselves, they may focus the same critical rigor onto their children's bodies. Identifying and exploring the impact of these family values and belief structures can be the first step. It can help to consider what factors may have influenced these (potentially) generational beliefs and disentangle the desire for acceptance from the drive for a certain size. Once we do this, we can start to more directly address the longings for connection that are attempting to resolve through our body.

Client Spotlight: Sporty Girlfriends

Josh lived in a larger body and had grown up in a family where thinness and "healthy eating" were of great value. He enjoyed reading and listening to music and felt like an outsider in a family of fitness-focused extroverts. As he got older, Josh saw the pitfalls of their constant quest for body mastery and the way it ran their lives. At the same time, he felt invisible to them.

Josh made friends easily and had a number of long-term girlfriends in high school. He observed that his parents were more interested and engaged with him when he was dating athletic women. Initially he found himself thinking that by dating attractive, sporty women "it might make my body a little more tolerable to them." Once Josh realized he had unconsciously been pursuing connection with his family by choosing girlfriends they had things in common with, it made more room for his preferences when it came to the qualities he wanted in a romantic partner.

The Triple Whammy

What if the subculture we have chosen to be a part of (and which may serve as a proxy for the family that wasn't able to meet our needs) has body size or shape requirements? And to complicate things further if we did not feel a sense of belonging in our family of origin, we may be tempted to shapeshift to gain acceptance into a culture we find ourselves drawn to or part of. We call that the triple whammy of body image belonging.

While families of origin can have strong values placed on specific body sizes, many subcultures also convey messages about body shape and size. Some examples of cultures that may have specific body types as part of their overt or covert requirements for belonging are: certain sports, professions, fitness communities, etc. There is value in getting clear on which messages come from each culture. Making these influences visible allows us to get curious as to what choices we have in response to them.

Exercise 5.5 Shapeshifted vs Authentic

We have talked about all the ways we change ourselves for the sake of acceptance and connection. Let's illustrate the differences between your shapeshifted and authentic puzzle pieces.

*We invite you to draw your **shapeshifted** puzzle piece. Write three to five adjectives that describe your shapeshifted personality patterns.*

1. _____ 2. _____ 3. _____ 4. _____ 5. _____

Example:

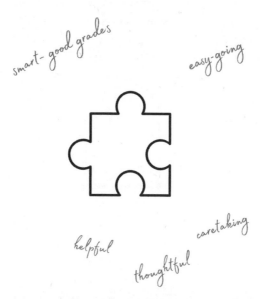

smart – good grades

easy-going

helpful

thoughtful

caretaking

Your turn:

Now try this again with a more authentic representation of your puzzle piece.

*Write three to five adjectives that describe your **authentic** personality and preferences to help you connect with who you are without shapeshifting.*

1. _____ 2. _____ 3. _____ 4. _____ 5. _____

*Draw the shape of your **authentic** puzzle piece here (space below) or find another way to express your authentic nature with art, dance, or music.*

Example:

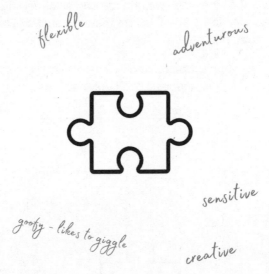

flexible   adventurous

sensitive

goofy – likes to giggle   creative

Your turn:

Exercise 5.6 The Relational Mirror: A Reflection Practice

In your early mirroring, you didn't have any control over who mirrored you or what they mirrored back. Your body image has been trying to help you compensate for any unskilled, inaccurate or impaired early mirroring you received. In its makeshift way, your body image has been trying to create the belonging and safety you longed for in your relationships.

The goal of this exercise is to build more awareness around how different relationships make you and your body feel. This insight will help you see which relationships may be triggering your urge to shapeshift and ultimately give you more choice in how you navigate your relationships. Pick a relationship that doesn't always leave you feeling good in your skin and fill out the following prompts.

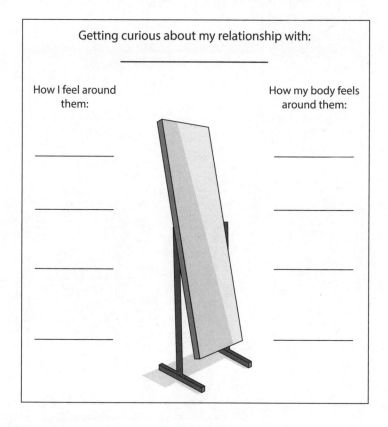

Getting curious about my relationship with:

_____

How I feel around them:

_____

_____

_____

_____

How my body feels around them:

_____

_____

_____

_____

Are there ways you shapeshift your emotions or behaviors in this relationship?

_____

_____

How can you prepare for potential BBIMs when you do spend time with this person?

_____

_____

Is there anything you can do to diminish the amount of time you spend in front of your negative relational mirrors?

_____

_____

Now pick a relationship that has a positive impact on you or leaves you feeling comfortable/good/connected:

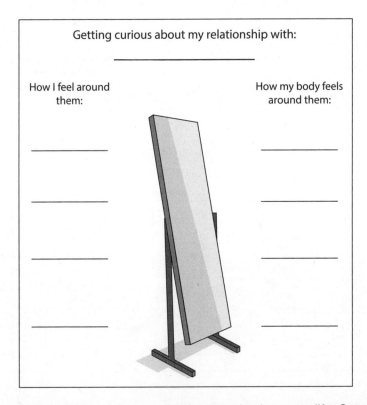

Getting curious about my relationship with:

_____

How I feel around them:

How my body feels around them:

Start to build this relational mirror reflection practice into your life. Get curious about how you, your body and your body image feel in response to various relationships. You can use this insight to gain clarity about which relationships you invest in and which ones you may need to be more resourced for. Even if you can't avoid certain people, you will be able to anticipate and prepare for potential BBIMs.

Bless the truth inside you

The messy, inconvenient, vulnerable truth

Pushing itself up to be revealed like a sprouting seed

Bless its origin, deep within the unique map of you

Bless its uncomfortable journey

*Bless the old messages that have instructed it to stay
hidden—Believing that would keep you safe.*

*Bless the truth within you: its life, its importance
and its possibility.*

6 | Decoding
Learning to Speak Body Image

"There is more wisdom in your body than in your deepest philosophy."

Nietzsche

Learning to decode sounds like you're training to be a secret agent, doesn't it? Well, you are on a very important mission, and you are the only one on this planet who has access to the vital information you need to succeed. Your mission is to lead a fuller, richer, more emotionally-satisfying life. Decoding is a crucial element of the BodySelf process. If we don't learn how to understand what our body image is trying to tell us, then we don't get the opportunity to take care of the parts of us for which our body image is speaking. In this chapter we are going to break down the steps needed to dialogue with your body image in a new way.

"What is Happening in My Body" Becomes "How I Feel About My Body"

Remember when we talked about how we can wake up feeling pretty good about how we look and by lunchtime we hate what we see in the mirror? Or those moments when it feels like some part of our body, or perhaps all of it, is growing or changing before our eyes? While it could be hormones or humidity, it is much more likely that over the course of our day, something has shaken us up emotionally and our body image is communicating that. Decoding gives us an opportunity to interview our body image, to ask it for a "printout" and then interpret what it is actually saying. Decoding can apply to these immediate spikes in negative body image, and it can also offer insights in looking at more long-standing critical belief patterns we have had about our body, all those unspoken emotions and sensations that are inside us waiting to be heard and understood.

The sensations we feel in our body are important in the decoding process. These sensations, particularly the ones in the regular rotation in our body image dialogue, are clues that can help us understand what our body image is saying. Here are a few examples of how this mash-up of emotions, sensations and body image can sound:

- My droopy arm skin feels like it's going to fall off.
- My thighs feel like stuffed sausages that are about to burst.
- My torso feels thick and my back fat is vibrating.
- My shoulders are hulkish, it feels like they are taking over my body.
- My stomach feels so round and full but empty.

Here is a decoding mini-session to give you a chance to see how decoding can sound in real time and how sensations fit into the process.

Decoding Mini-session: Overtaking Me

BodySelf: Hi Dylan, how are you feeling today?

Dylan: *I feel awful in my body, like I just can't be in it. It feels so massive, like it's overtaking me.*

BodySelf: Do you have a sense of when your body image shifted, when you started to feel so negatively towards your body?

Dylan: *I went home last weekend to see my mom, and it was really hard. Being around her brings up so much.*

BodySelf: That is good information. Would it be OK if we circled back to your body image and wrote down the words that you were using to describe how it felt to be home last weekend? I think it might help us understand why you feel so awful in your body right now.

Dylan: *Sure ... Sigh. It's so hard being there, and before I know it, I just start to feel like shit about myself.*

BodySelf: That makes so much sense. If you can, just try to speak on your body image's behalf. Like if it had the floor, what would it say?

Dylan: *OK ... I can't be in this body, it feels impossible. Like there is just too much of it—it is massive. And it keeps growing and changing, I don't feel like myself, and I am so uncomfortable in my own skin.*

BodySelf: Great. Let's pause for a second and take the time to write down what you are saying so we can really appreciate and examine your word choices:

- "I just can't be in it. It feels so massive, like it's overtaking me."
- "I can't be in this body, it feels impossible. Like there is just too much of it."
- "It keeps growing and changing, I don't feel like myself."
- "Uncomfortable in my skin."

What are you noticing as you see those words?

Dylan: *Woah, that is exactly how I feel when I am there, at my mom's house! She is taking me over. She is too much! Her mood keeps changing and I can't keep up. It's impossible to be around her and not feel so confused. I stop knowing who I am and what is true for me because I am trying to either protect myself from what she is saying or find a way to please her.*

BodySelf: See what else you are noticing as you see those words?

Dylan: *Overtaking—yeah, that is how it feels … like she is overtaking me, and I don't want to be there anymore. I think I don't want to be in my body, but I think the truth is, I don't want to be in that house … It feels impossible to be there and stay connected to myself.*

BodySelf: What do you think your body image might be trying to tell you, Dylan?

Dylan: *I just can't have the same conversation with her again and again. I can't open up my heart anymore. I can't try again and be disappointed. It's just too hard. I don't know what I am going to do next, but I see how negatively impacted I am by her. I can't imagine actually doing it … but I need to figure out how I can take some space from the relationship.*

Dylan's specific discomfort in his body provided valuable clues about how uncomfortable he felt in his current relationship with his mom. When Dylan listened to the specific words he used to describe the sensations, he had access to much more clarity about how he was feeling in his relationship with her. Now, let's dig into learning the Decoding Steps we used above.

> *"The universe buries strange jewels deep within us all, and then stands back to see if we can find them."*
>
> Elizabeth Gilbert

Decoding Step 1: What's the Dialogue?

To translate our body image, we need to get an accurate transcript of what our body image is saying. The first step is getting the "data" by asking the right questions and writing down the answers. This step might feel simple, but putting into words what our body image is saying to us can feel quite vulnerable. We rarely say these words out loud, and if we do, they are often paired with sarcasm or shame. So please offer yourself some extra compassion as you invite your body image to communicate with you. This is a great time to grab that sensation list from Chapter 3 and see if any of the words help you articulate what you are feeling.

Exercise 6.1 Discovering Your Dialogue

Here are some suggestions to guide you in accessing your decoding transcript and getting your body image dialogue on the page. We invite you to use these questions or feel free to create some of your own.

What are the thoughts that you are having about your body right now?

_____

_____

What are the phrases that keep going through your head about your body?

_____

_____

What are the beliefs you have about your body/appearance right now?

_____

_____

What are the sensations that you are experiencing in your body right now?

_____

_____

What is the body "fix" that feels compelling right now?

_____

_____

What do you hope the "fix" will give you that you don't have right now?

_____

_____

Example:

What are the thoughts that you are having about your body right now?

My body looks like a slug, like I am just soft and shapeless.

What are the phrases that keep going through your head about your body?

I have no definition, everything about my body is soft and squishy.

What are the beliefs you have about your body/appearance right now?

My body is boring, it has no real shape.

What are the sensations that you are experiencing in your body right now?

It feels like my body is melting, like it's losing its shape and energy.

What is the body "fix" that feels compelling right now?

I need to be stronger, more toned with more defined edges.

What do you hope the "fix" will give you?

I would stand out more. People would notice me and want to get to know me.

Now that you have your dialogue, let's practice taking the judgment out.

Decoding Step 2: Remove the Judgment

What happens if we separate out the negativity from our body image dialogue? What remains? Earlier in the book we taught you about non-judgment, curiosity and compassion. When you are decoding, "removing the judgment" is like using a black light in a dark room; it enables you to see things that you might not see with the naked eye. Here are some examples of judgmental body criticism, and how with some judgment removal, we can access more nuanced truth about ourselves.

- "My legs aren't toned or firm enough." **If we take the judgment out:** *I would like legs that are more toned and firm. I want to have a strong physical presence.*

- "I feel big and out of place." **If we take the judgment out:** *There is something about me that feels uncomfortably large and doesn't fit in with the other people around me.*

- "My butt is so flat and boring." **If we take the judgment out:** *My butt is smaller than the big trendy butts that seem to be dancing all the time. I worry that people wont notice me.*

- "I look awful in dresses, they never feel like they fit right. I must just have the wrong body." **If we take the judgment out:** *I feel uncomfortable in dresses. I have a short torso and it always feels like I have a skirt around my ribs. I just feel so much more confident in pants.*

- "I need to push myself harder and go to the gym more. Maybe then I would get more responses on my dating app." **If we take the judgment out:** *I don't really like dating and I keep telling myself if I went to the gym more often, then all the people I like would like me back.*

Decoding Step 3: Identify Your Key Words and Phrases

There is valuable information embedded in the language you use about your body. Let's get out a magnifying glass to look for common words, phrases and themes when you think about and describe your body (especially the parts that you are unhappy with and want to change). Pay special attention to:

- Words and phrases that you say or think often
- Words that carry an emotional charge
- Adjectives and sensations
- Anything that sounds like it might be a descriptor of underlying emotions, dilemmas or conflicts

There is no template for the associations between our body image and our truth. Decoding is a personal process unique to each individual and each BBIM. The interpretation of "undefined legs" or "poofy stomach" or "bulky shoulders" will mean different things for different people. This is why you are the only one who can decode your body image (though others can most certainly accompany you in the process). Taking our words and disentangling them from our judgment can make it easier to find what word clues to investigate.

Here is an example from Exercise 6.1:

What are the thoughts that you are having about your body right now?

My body looks like a <u>slug</u>, like I am just <u>soft and shapeless.</u>

What are the phrases that keep going through your head about your body?

I have <u>no definition</u>, everything about my body is <u>soft and squishy</u>.

What are the beliefs you have about your body/appearance right now?

My body is <u>boring</u>, it has <u>no real shape</u>.

What are the sensations that you are experiencing in your body right now?

It feels like my body is <u>melting</u>, like it's <u>losing its energy</u>.

What is the body "fix" that feels compelling right now?

I need to be <u>stronger, more toned</u> with more <u>defined edges</u>.

What do you hope the "fix" will give you that you don't have right now?

People would see me differently. I'd <u>stand out</u> more. I would be more <u>noticeable</u>.

Exercise 6.2 Find Your Key Words

What words or phrases stood out in your dialogue from exercise 6.1?

_____

_____

What words or phrases carried a charge?

_____

_____

What words or phrases are ones you use often?

_____

_____

Client Spotlight: Everything is Just Hanging Out

After years of yearning and hesitation, Sam finally found the courage to sign up for a week-long writing retreat. She had a wonderful experience and shared far more of her writing than she had anticipated, even offering to volunteer to have her short story workshopped by the entire group.

As she was driving home, she was irritated to find herself feeling uncomfortable in her skin and focused on her stomach. It felt to her like "everything was hanging out," that she "wasn't contained." Did she eat too much at the meals? Did she not go on enough walks? She had been to a BodySelf workshop recently and knew these negative thoughts were a cue to get curious. Her body image was trying to tell her something.

When she got home, Sam wrote about this experience with her body. She realized that standing up in the workshop and sharing her story left her feeling quite vulnerable. She grew up in a family of big forceful personalities, and she had adapted by keeping her needs small.

At the retreat, sharing in a large group and asking for feedback was a bold step in a new direction. She had "put it all out there" in a wonderful, but unfamiliar way with people she had only just met.

> She was able to embrace how much courage it took for her to go to the workshop and how brave she had been to "put herself out there" in these new ways. Sam was amazed by how clearly her body was speaking to her, that it was signaling feelings of excitement and vulnerability that were important and needed space to be processed. She *did* "let everything hang out" and was proud of herself for doing it.

We can, like the writer Matt Haig suggests, think of our words as "seeds" and use "language (as) a way back to life." Simply focusing on the body part where the intense feelings reside can be a starting point for decoding.

Decoding Step 4: Interpret Your Words

Let's recap the decoding steps we have learned so far before we introduce the final one.

- **Step 1** is to write out the dialogue.
- **Step 2** removing the judgment.
- **Step 3** is to find your key words.
- **Step 4** is attuning to the language about your body, and then investigating where these descriptors might apply to your broader life. This inquiry is at the heart of turning your body image inside-out.

Take a look at your words from Exercise 6.2 and let's explore how these words may have similarities to aspects of your life. Choose the word that stands out to you, whether it's one you say often or when you read your answers evokes the strongest emotional response. Let's say a word that you use often to describe your body is *jiggly*. First, come up with a few words similar to *jiggly* and see if any of them resonate even more. For example, alternate words to *jiggly* are: *restless, shaky, squirmy, fidgety*. Maybe the word *restless* feels like a better fit. Here is an example exploring key words:

Example:

- My keyword is *jiggly*
- Similar words are: *restless, shaky, squirmy, fidgety*
- What word resonates the most? *restless*

Follow up questions:

- Where else outside of my body do things feel *restless*?

- Are there any areas of my life where things feel *restless*?
- Do I feel like I am showing up *restless* in any particular area of my life?

It can also be helpful to think about opposing words. There may be an area of your life that you wish was the opposite of *restless*, and more *firm, stable, reliable* or *settled*. Similarly, see which of these words resonates most. Here is an example of exploring opposing words:

- My word is *restless*.
- Opposite words are *firm, stable, reliable or settled*.
- The word that most resonates of all of these is *stable*.
- If my life were more *stable*, I would feel *calm and confident*.
- Are there any areas of my life where I long for things to feel more *stable*?
- Does *stable* capture how I want to feel about some aspect of my life?

Exercise 6.3 Leaning into Your Words

Here are some questions to help you find the connection between your body image key words and the broader context of your life.

My word is _____

Similar words are _____, _____ *and* _____

The word that most resonates for me is _____

Where else outside of my body do things feel _____?

Do I feel like I am showing up _____ *in any particular area of my life?*

Are there any areas of my life where things feel _____?

My opposing words are _____, _____ *and* _____

The opposing word that most resonates for me is _____

If my life were more _____, *I would feel more* _____

Are there any areas of my life where I long for things to feel more _____?

_____

Does _____ *capture how I want to feel about some aspect of my life?*

_____

Here is a mini-session to demonstrate how this process of exploring your key words can sound in a dialogue. We have bolded the words and phrases that stand out and appear to be clues about what Sarafina's body image dialogue is saying.

Mini Decoding Session: Not What I Need it to Be

BodySelf: Hi. How are you feeling coming in today?

Sarafina: *Meh, pretty low. It has been a shitty two weeks since I last saw you. I don't want to deal with anything. I feel so unsettled. All of my energy is being taken up by my body image.*

BodySelf: Tell me more, what are you noticing?

Sarafina: *I don't have any clothes that I like. I want to empty my closet completely. Dressing for work is torture—nothing looks good.* **Nothing makes me feel like myself.** *I just want to scream. I feel angry that I have this critical part that takes up so much space and is always saying I'm* **not good enough.**

BodySelf: It sounds like a lot of self-criticism is coming up as you're getting dressed for work and ready for your day. How are you feeling in other parts of your day?

Sarafina: *Ugggh, I hate my new job. My new boss is so checked out. She says she sees how she can help me advance beyond this boring introductory role but has no time to actually help get me there. I feel like there is* **no real plan** *for me and that leaves me being everyone's administrative support. I feel frustrated and bored and lonely. I thought I was chosen by this cool company where I could work my way up but my role and trajectory are totally* **undefined and unclear.** *It makes me feel like a failure.*

BodySelf: What feels hardest about all of this?

Sarafina: *It is hard to know what to trust. I feel so confused. What I was told when I took the position, what advancement was possible and how I would be utilized, is soooo different from the reality of my job.*

BodySelf: If it is OK with you, I would like to circle back to what is going on between you and your closet.

Sarafina: *Sure. Well, I need to do something because I want to get rid of everything in my closet. It feels like* **nothing fits. I don't fit.** *I don't want to wear anything to work because I don't actually want to be there. My clothes* **don't look right** *on my body. My body feels different and wrong. I am not what this job wants me to be.*

BodySelf: I wonder if you take out the self-criticism, and judgment, what is left in what you are saying?

Sarafina: *[silence, some tears]*

Bodyself: Sarafina, given what we have explored so far, what is more clear to you?

Sarafina: *This job is* **not what I need it to be.**

> **BodySelf:** It sounds like it is really hard to figure out what to wear to a job that *isn't a fit for you*. And that given how you are being managed, anyone would have a hard time feeling like they were a fit for this job. What I hear you saying is, that *nothing in your closet works because the job doesn't work*.
>
> **Sarafina:** *[More tears, a very big sigh]*

> *"When you write your truth, it is a love offering to the world because it helps us feel braver and less alone."*
>
> Glennon Doyle

Exercise 6.4 Your Mini Decoding Session

Now, you give decoding a try. Think of a recent or recurring BBIM …

BodySelf: Hi. How are you feeling today?

You: _____

BodySelf: Tell me more, what are you noticing about your body image?

You: _____

BodySelf: It sounds like a lot of self-criticism is coming up around. How are you feeling in other parts of your life?

You: _____

BodySelf: Tell me more, what else?

BodySelf: What feels hardest about these challenges in your life?

You: _____

BodySelf: Can you go back and highlight any words about your body or body image that stand out to you or have extra charge?

You: These words are: _____

BodySelf: How might these words or phrases be related to something that is going on more broadly?

You: Well, the words _____ *I think relate to* _____

_____

BodySelf: Wonderful decoding. Can you bring some compassion to how you are feeling and what your body image is trying to communicate?

You: I have compassion for how hard _____ *feels to me. I appreciate that my body image is trying to tell me* _____

_____

Decoding a Specific Body Part

Often the size or shape of a certain body part comes to hold feelings or meaning. Exploring the story of what that part of the body "holds" can reveal a deeper dilemma or longing inside. It can be helpful to get curious about what these body parts have come to represent.

Here are some examples:

- Essie associated wide hips with the women on her mother's side of the family, whom she had never felt comfortable around growing up. Her maternal relatives were opinionated, forceful, and not interested in whether they were making others uncomfortable. Essie had a much quieter, softer presence and attuned to others easily. For Essie, her naturally wider hips became paired with fears of being bossy and misattuned to others. She was afraid of taking up too much space in a room like her aunts and focused endless hours exercising chasing slimmer hips.

- Ivy had grown up with a very timid mother and depressed father, both of whom seemed to move through the world slumped over. Ivy wanted to lead a life of intention and impact. By standing tall and having a strong presence, she felt she could distinguish herself from her parents. Because she so deeply wanted to be different, she often overtrained her arms and shoulders to the point of injury. Her commitment to her upper body strength had become coupled with avoiding the sorrow and fragility she saw in her parents.

Once we start to discover that parts of our body may have come to represent our fears, our hopes or our longings, we have an opportunity to get to know them.

Client Spotlight: Sad Legs

In her weekly body image group, Sylvi described feeling really focused on her legs and how critical she was feeling toward them. She also shared with the group that she felt really shaken after receiving a judgmental email from her dad. When the group leader asked if Sylvi might be able to speak for her legs and see what they might want her to know, Sylvi knew right away. "I have sad legs. They are pulling me down, like I just want to crumple."

One of the other members chimed in, "Oh my gosh, I know exactly what you are talking about, I have 'sad legs' sometimes too!"

Sylvi added, "It's like they are my little scorekeepers, they have been with me all along. Now, I know what they are saying and why they are saying it. I have felt sad legs so many times in my life, and it always turned into feeling like there was something wrong with them, that I should go for a run or do something to make them better. I just didn't have the words to describe what I was actually feeling. Now I can listen and they can have the floor! Sometimes a run does help, but other times my 'sad legs' just need me to be gentle with them and curl up under a cozy blanket and rest."

Exercise 6.5 Decoding Mad Lib

Pick a body part that you feel critical of and/or wish were different (see example below):

My belief about my _____ *is that* _____

What this belief says about me is that I am _____

If I didn't have this/these _____ *I would be* _____

If I didn't have this/these _____ *my life would be* _____

Example:

For Essie (above)

My belief about my hips *is that they are* too wide.

What this belief says about me is that I am pushy, take up a lot of space and make others uncomfortable.

If I didn't have this/these wide hips *I would be* more likable.

If I didn't have this/these hips *my life would be* more free.

Recap: The Four Decoding Steps

Step 1 Write out your inner body image dialogue.

Step 2 Remove the judgment.

Step 3 Find your key words.

Step 4 Refine your words and explore where your body image language might apply to your broader life.

Bless your decoding mission, you are the only one in the entire world who can lead this investigation.

May you recognize the messages your body is holding.

And learn the sacred language of your wounds and your wants.

May you listen well and find those with whom to share what you hear.

May laughter be invited into the task of uncovering your deeper truth.

And the ribbons of translation wrap you in new possibilities for your relationship with yourself.

7 | I'll Have What They're Having
Decoding Jealousy

"Jealousy can be a beautiful opportunity to deepen our awareness of what we want and who we are."

Joli Hamilton

Othello called jealousy the "green-eyed monster" who mocks. We all know that feeling, when someone catches our eye because they are attractive or especially put together. It could be at a party, at the gym, in the grocery store or just walking down the street. We have a hard time not staring at them. Something in us has been awakened. Quickly and often unconsciously, we make all sorts of inferences; our mind spins a tale about who they are and what their lives are like. Within seconds, our initial experience of captivation transitions into comparing ourselves, and jealousy enters the scene. Something might tighten in our neck or drop in our belly, and before we know it, intrigue morphs into pain and hopelessness.

Our brains are wired for jealousy. Evolutionary psychologists believe that jealousy evolved to help us protect our partnerships, our bond with our mates. Although this was all well and good when we lived in a small tribe, clan or village, it has entirely different repercussions in a world that constantly bombards us with images of idealized bodies on billboards, in magazines, and of course, social media—oh boy, social media! With no training or tools, we're expected to metabolize thousands of images and the complex feelings they may inspire. Rather than push them away, we want to teach you to lean into these complicated feelings of jealousy and see what you learn.

Typically, jealousy is associated with negativity and most of us have carried the bias that it's something we "shouldn't" feel. Instead, we invite you to step through that daunting door and see what rich and vital information lives on the other side. Like so many other aspects of the BodySelf, by bringing curiosity to the table we create an opportunity for deeper self-discovery. The road from jealousy to alignment isn't very long, you just need curiosity to get there.

There are long-held beliefs in the body image field that the best way to heal negative body image is to teach clients to shift from a "comparing" mindset to one of self-love and acceptance. When talking with other practitioners about body image work, we often hear comments like, "My client is always comparing herself to other people and I keep trying to direct her towards positive aspects of herself." We honor the goal of that perspective and our "inside out" approach asks, "What can be *uncovered* in our jealousy?"

Client Spotlight: Michelle Obama Arms

Diya had been raised in a high-achieving, academically-focused family. Both of her parents were born and educated in India and had attained notable professional success. From early on, Diya felt a strong pressure to follow in her parents' footsteps and pursue a career in science. While both of her parents were respected and recognized professors, at home her father was verbally abusive towards her mom and spoke derogatively about women overall. It broke Diya's heart to see her brilliant mother cower around her father and she longed for her mom to stand up to her dad and leave the marriage.

Diya was obsessed with the physique of one of her female professors. When Diya described her professor, what she idealized most was her muscular "Michelle Obama arms." To Diya, her professor's strong arms represented so much more than defined biceps and triceps. She imagined her professor was not only an educator who had the strength to overcome the sexism and racism in the STEM world her own mother had faced, but also was in a loving partnership filled with safety and respect—just like Michelle Obama. Diya realized that her teacher's "Michelle Obama arms" represented what she wanted for herself and her mother, a successful career and a supportive partner.

From Skinny Girl to Pedestal Person

The inspiration for our approach to jealousy was born from a conversation at one of our early workshops. We asked attendees to describe what they were most fearful of in showing up that day. They had the expected worry about sharing their unspoken negative thoughts and beliefs with others. But an even greater anxiety, one we hadn't anticipated, was articulated when someone said, "the *skinny girl* might be here!" Everyone vigorously agreed. The group discovered that for each of them, the "*skinny girl*" was code for that person in the room who had the body that they had spent their lives trying to achieve. They described how much they feared facing some version of that person (and their body!). They expressed how confusing it was to feel both drawn to and resentful towards someone at the same time. They assumed that the presence of such a person could have only one outcome: self-judgment and a longing for something they could never have. Through this dialogue, it became clear that what people were reacting to was far deeper than an idealized body.

Because the term "Skinny Girl" echoes the negative influences of diet culture, we use the more inclusive and expansive term "Pedestal Person." In this chapter, we'll walk you through interviewing and deconstructing your "Pedestal Person," including the non-body-related elements of your envy. We have found that when we approach our jealousy with curiosity, we quickly discover that our jealousy isn't just about a perfect butt or bulging biceps, but the life that we imagine the owner of the butt and biceps to have.

Client Spotlight: Hip Hairdresser

Mari was jealous of her hairdresser, Anna. Maybe it's all that time staring in the mirror, but it seems like hairdressers have mastered their "look." Mari was focused on how comfortable Anna seemed in herself and her funky clothes. She imagined Anna easily putting together her outfits each morning while dancing around her colorful bedroom.

Growing up in a very conservative household where she was taught that there was one way to look and present oneself, Mari hadn't been allowed to experiment with her own clothing, make-up or hairstyle. Mari's mother had insisted she wear skirts and dresses and keep her hair in a low ponytail, emphasizing the importance of looking feminine and pretty but also not standing out. After doing the "Pedestal Person" exercise, it became clear to Mari that it wasn't just Anna's great sense of style she wanted, but the playfulness, ease and confidence she saw in Anna that she wanted more of. Mari had always wanted to wear flared jeans but thought they were too "cool" a look for her to pull off. After doing the "Pedestal" exercise, Mari took herself shopping and found bell-bottomed jeans that she loved. Anna initially incited envy in Mari; ultimately curiosity served as a portal to discover more about her own creative longings.

Decoding Jealousy: Working Outside-in

Mari's Pedestal Person was her hairdresser, what about yours? We want to teach you how to deconstruct your "Pedestal People." The process takes all the emotion that you put into comparison and redirects it through a lens of curiosity. It helps you shift from the isolation of self-judgment into a juicier conversation where you can truly examine what you want more of in your own life—and that typically extends far outside the realm of appearance. We propose that other people's outfits, accomplishments and lives serve as inspirations, not destinations. Your longings have so much to teach you about your own authenticity.

We have developed a three-step process to decode your jealousy.

1 **Get curious:** Jealousy is often experienced as self-criticism and desire intertwined. So what if we take a hold of the desire and follow where it leads? When we allow ourselves to connect to the longing and explore it, we bring to life the yearnings that our "Pedestal Person" inspires. In order for jealousy to teach rather than torment, we need to once again practice curiosity. First, clarify all that you admire and begin to wonder about what you see. *Mia looks so amazing in her flowy dress, I wish I were more like Mia! I wonder what it is about Mia and her dress that feels so compelling to me?*

2 **Turn it outside-in:** What if we were to shine a light that goes beyond their appearance and get curious about what we believe these physical attributes grant them in their life. What is the life we think they inhabit? How do you imagine it feels to look like, be like, live like them? What information does your envy offer you about what you long for? **Hint:** What makes your "Pedestal Person" powerful are the qualities and experiences YOU project onto them. *What is it that I like about Mia in her flowy dress? I imagine that in her flowy dress she has a flowy life. Her flowy life is full of relaxed dinners on the patio, lots of close friends and adventures in nature.*

3 **Own it:** Now this gets fun. Once you tease out what they've got that you want, you can start to play and experiment with how to bring more of that into your own life. *I imagine Mia's flowy life is full of relaxed dinners on the patio, lots of close friends and adventures in nature. Hmmm, I am really yearning for more close friendships, and I'd really like to plan some outings outside of the city. Where could I start?*

> *"There's always a porch light on to welcome us back. You just have to listen closely for the directions to lead you there."*
>
> Lalah Delia

Jealousy and Alignment

It might sound confusing to pair alignment and jealousy, but the details of our projections can bring us into more alignment with and connection to ourselves. Jealousy is our body's way of telling us that something about that other person resonates with us. The challenge is to not immediately focus on what we don't have, but to get curious and clear about what we are wanting more of. What we envy may be a feeling: ease, joy, connection. It may be a way of moving through the world: confidence, strength, alignment. It could be an experience: adventurous travel, romance or more time for creativity.

Client Spotlight: Pregnant Yogis

Annie was a bright, driven educator who never really felt like she was "enough" professionally. In parallel to her work life, she had always struggled with critical thoughts about her body and had been on a long and painful quest to look a certain way. It wasn't until she was pregnant that her "Pedestal Person" fully emerged and offered her some important insight.

During her pregnancy, Annie's ritual was to eat dinner at the salad bar at Whole Foods before her 6 pm therapy appointment. She began each therapy session by describing a group of pregnant women she saw leaving their prenatal yoga class every Tuesday night and getting salads while Annie was eating her dinner. She longed to look more like them and felt "schlumpy" and "enormous" in comparison. They seemed to move with great ease in their "fit" pregnant bodies as Annie watched them float from the beans to the feta, and she imagined they felt comfortable in their skin and loved watching their bellies grow.

This was a far cry from the experience Annie was having in her own pregnancy, which involved acute nausea, extreme fatigue and very little energy for exercise or even gentle movement. She longed for the confidence and excitement she imagined these pregnant power yoga women were feeling. As she unpacked her fantasies of what it was like to live in their bodies rather than her own, she connected to her grief and sadness about how incredibly hard her pregnancy had been and how disconnected she felt from her body and her pre-pregnancy life. Ultimately it was helpful for Annie to give voice to her experience and to honor the parts of her that felt like they couldn't or shouldn't feel this way. When she was able to express her grief and overwhelm, her body focus shifted significantly and she started to think about what other supports she needed during her pregnancy.

"We're so lucky that flowers don't hold themselves back because other flowers are already blooming."

Emily McDowell

Exercise 7.1 Pedestal Person

Your turn: Who is *your* Pedestal Person?

Uncovering your Pedestal Person can help you shrink the distance between envy and your own aliveness. Following your curiosity can help you access how you want to feel in your life and in your body. Let's meet *the person you idealize* and get curious about what they have to teach you.

Who sparks jealousy in you? They may be a colleague at work or someone you routinely visit on your social media feed. They may have similarities to you or be a different gender, race or age.

Pedestal Person: _____

Get curious: First, clarify all that you admire about their appearance. How would you describe this person? Be as detailed as you can. Some examples include: stylish, sporty, broad shoulders, long legs, smooth skin, thick hair, etc. If you run out of space, you can add your notes to a journal or notebook.

_____

_____

Go outside-in: Let's get curious about what you think these physical attributes grant them in their life. How do you imagine it feels to look like, be like, live like them? Answer any of the below questions you are drawn to:

What do you like about how they look?

_____

_____

However you answered above, what do you imagine this physical quality or attribute allows them to do/gives them access to?

_____

_____

How do they feel about themselves and how did they arrive there?

_____

_____

How do they spend their time and money? What does a typical day look like for them?

_____

_____

What type of impact do they have on others?

_____

_____

How do other people treat them and respond to them?

_____

_____

Who is their community or chosen family?

_____

_____

How do they express themselves creatively?

_____

_____

What are you drawn to in their lifestyle? Do they like to travel or are they more into nesting?

_____

_____

Own it: *Once you tease out what they have that you want, you can experiment with how to bring more of that into your own life. Identify the characteristic you feel most drawn to in your Pedestal Person by looking over the answers above and circle characteristics or aspects of their life that you feel most aligned with.*

The quality/trait/life circumstances that I circled above are:

_____

_____

_____

Now let's answer some additional questions about your research. You can do this with as many qualities as you like.

The quality/trait/life circumstance that I circled above is:

_____

If I were to have more _____ *in my life, one small step
I could take would be:*

_____

Imagine taking that step. How do you think that would make you feel?

_____

_____

What limiting beliefs might get in the way of you taking that small step?

_____

_____

What kind of support might help?

_____

_____

Example:

The quality/trait/life circumstance that I circled above is:

More freedom.

If I were to have more freedom in my life, one small step I could take would be:

Saying no to spending a holiday with my family of origin and going away with friends instead.

Imagine taking that step. How do you think that would make you feel?

Liberated, adventurous, guilty.

What limiting beliefs might get in the way of you taking that small step?

That I should choose what makes them happy over my own desires.

What kind of support might help?

My friends and my cousin who also does his own thing on holidays sometimes.

Now that you have gone through the steps of decoding your jealousy, we hope you can use curiosity next time the green-eyed monster strikes!

Bless the jealous parts in you, may you meet them with an outstretched hand.

Bless the Green-Eyed Monster, for they are carrying an important message.

Do not fear their monster growls, but rather see the mirror in their eye—reflecting back more of who you are.

8 | Cracking the Clothing Code

"Style is the only thing you can't buy. It's not in a shopping bag, a label, or a price tag. It's something reflected from our soul to the outside world."

Alber Elbaz

Clothing can save the day when we find an outfit we love for an exciting event or bring us to our knees when the seventh pair of jeans we have tried on don't fit the way we had hoped. Clothing is like a second skin. It is an extension of body image, offering us another way to access what needs to be understood, expressed or resourced. Getting dressed is something we do every day. For these reasons, we can discover and align more with ourselves by exploring our relationship with clothing. It gives us a chance to notice what happens inside of us when we are choosing what to wear for work, a date, a family wedding or a job interview. Learning how to dialogue with our thoughts and feelings about our clothes can guide us more skillfully through our most challenging wardrobe dilemmas. We are going to teach you how to crack the clothing code so that you can create a more connected conversation with your clothes, your closet and yourself.

Clothing is polarizing and powerful—it invites us to express ourselves and can feel like a measure of our worth. Our clothing choices tell the world about us and our story. Ask anyone why they love or hate what they are wearing, and they will have something to say. Clothing elicits memories and represents experiences and chapters of our lives. Discarding an item might help us shed an aspect of ourselves we have outgrown and getting something new might express an evolving truth about who we are becoming. Often, something is being expressed emotionally through our interpretation of how we look in our clothes. We often quickly jump to, "I look terrible," or "this outfit is lame," or "nothing looks good on me today." But this sentiment might be trying to communicate something else. With all of these dimensions, it's no wonder simply choosing a shirt to wear to an event can be paralyzing if we aren't sure who or what we want to project to the people we will see there. How can we make our relationship to our clothing less fraught and more joyful?

In this chapter we will explore:

- How our history with shopping, clothing and getting dressed can impact our current relationship to clothing.
- How to use curiosity and creativity to explore our sensory and emotional experiences of clothing.
- How to decode our clothing dilemmas.
- How to develop a more collaborative relationship with our closet.

Clothing can be:

- A way to measure ourselves, to evaluate and assess our body.
- A boundary.
- A way to hide or protect ourselves.
- A way to try to stand out or fit in.
- A way to experiment with our identity.
- A way to resource ourselves.
- A way to express ourselves.

Clothing History

Much like with body image, many factors play into our relationship with clothing. Our early experiences of getting dressed and going shopping can strongly affect how we feel in our clothes. We may have received messaging, stated or unstated, about our worth based on how our caregivers handled the process of dressing us. We invite you to get curious about these influences.

Client Spotlight: One Size Smaller

Alison had always wanted to be a cheerleader and spent most of her afternoons in grade school teaching herself the tricks she saw at high school football games. She was thrilled to make the cheerleading team when she was in junior high and over the moon when her high school squad made it to the state finals.

Growing up, Alison's mom had been critical of both her own weight and Alison's. Whenever they went clothes shopping together, it was a painful experience. Her mom often chose clothes for Alison that she deemed "flattering"—dark slacks and nothing with horizontal stripes or bright colors that would draw attention to her midsection. Alison loved vivid colors and prints and always left these shopping trips feeling like she was in the wrong body and consequently in the wrong clothes.

When Alison's mom took her to get fitted for her state finals uniform, she insisted they get it one size smaller, assuring Alison the size would be a "motivator" for weight loss. Alison felt so proud of how hard she had worked all these years to get to this competition and was devastated that her mom still felt she was in the wrong body.

It took her years to re-evaluate this early messaging and feel comfortable in her own skin. Now, she is committed to letting go of pieces of clothing that don't feel right, inside or out, and takes great care in choosing things that "fit" her natural shape in whatever color she fancies.

This is a story we have heard many times over, how someone else's attachment to *their* size becomes their attachment to *our* size. In our early lives, the people who take us shopping and dress us can have a huge impact on our experience of clothing and our bodies. Think about who took you shopping and what that experience was like. Did you know what clothing you were drawn to? How did the person who took you shopping respond? Take a moment to think about the start of your clothing story, and what influences shaped it.

Exercise 8.1 Clothing History

this left me feeling
- - - - - - - - -
- - - - - - - - -
- - - - - - - - -
- - - - - - - - -

Experience: Who took you shopping as a kid? Are there any experiences that stand out to you?

_____

_____

_____

_____

Descriptors: If so, what are three descriptors that capture how these experiences left you feeling?

_____

_____

Current belief: Are there any beliefs or struggles from these early experiences that still accompany you on your shopping trips?

_____

_____

Example:

Experience: Who took you shopping as a kid? Are there any experiences that stand out to you?

When I went shopping with my dad, it was an arduous experience. It took me forever to find something I liked at all, and when I did he would always say it was too expensive. We rarely bought anything that wasn't practical and almost ways ended up with another pair of plain, ugly jeans and a boring button-down.

Descriptors: If so, what are three descriptors that capture how these experiences left you feeling?

Not valuable, rejected, frustrated

Current belief: Are there any beliefs or struggles from these early experiences that still accompany you on your shopping trips?

Finding things that I like often takes time. I used to feel terribly guilty when I bought things that were a little pricier than normal. Now I am able to trust myself and buy fewer things that I adore.

Clothing is Containing

Clothing can offer a sense of safety, a way to calm or regulate ourselves when we feel overwhelmed. Most of us can relate to having clothing in our closet that we hang onto even though it isn't in the regular rotation. We may have an article of clothing that we have kept as a way to measure ourselves. It may represent a certain size, identity or longing. We may turn to this article of clothing when we need reassurance or grounding.

Client Spotlight: The Skirt that Kept Me Safe

Cass had grown up in a home with two unhappily married parents and as an only child had never felt a sense of belonging in her small disconnected family. As a happily married mom and successful executive in her fifties, Cass was warm and enthusiastic. She had the kind of energy that led you to believe that she was comfortable in any setting. She had navigated some body image and disordered eating patterns in her adolescence but, as an adult, she felt committed to body acceptance and as a rule, she did not have any scales in her home.

Yet, in the corner of her walk-in closet was a skirt she had kept for almost four decades. The skirt had stayed with Cass through every move and every closet clean-out. In times of stress, she would take this skirt out and try it on. She assumed that keeping it and trying it on at random times had been a way to track her body, and she had never actually explored why this skirt was so sacred to her. When menopause prompted Cass to work with a nutritionist, she was able to explore and discover the meaning of the skirt. Cass had worn it many times in the early months of dating her wife, Olivia. She realized that being able to fit into the skirt helped her access the feelings of comfort and safety she had first felt with her wife. Over time, Cass was able to bring more curiosity to when and why "the skirt" came out for fittings. She also started to build in nurturing rituals and tools that offered security and reassurance when she had the urge to try it on.

Cass's story captures the essence of how our relationship to a piece of clothing may serve a function beyond our image. Our job is to get curious about what parts of ourselves these pieces of clothing are tending to. Decoding a charged relationship with a certain piece of clothing can offer insight about what we are craving in our lives or what we want to express. For example, if we are habitually using a piece of clothing as a measuring tool, we can examine what is happening in the moments we are drawn to "measure" ourselves. Or if we are drawn to a particular piece of clothing, like a bright red blazer, every time we are anticipating a meeting where we think our voice will be stifled, this red blazer might be trying to speak for us and saying, "Listen to me!"

Did you ever think you would have a conversation with your pants? We do it all the time. Here is an example of what we can learn when we dialogue with charged clothing.

Mini Clothing Decoding Session: The Power of the Pants

Jamie: *I have been trying to clean out my closet before I move. I have so many clothes from different chapters of my life. It's been easy to let go of some of my dresses and tops, but I just can't seem to let go of any of my pants. Whenever I try to put them in the giveaway pile, I feel panicked.*

BodySelf: Would you be open to having a conversation with those pants? Maybe they can help you understand why they are so resistant to change.

Jamie: *I just don't understand, and I would really like to.*

BodySelf: Great, I am going to ask you some questions and I would like you to answer as if you are "Jamie's pants." Jamie's pants, can you help us understand why you are so afraid of Jamie letting you go? Can you tell us more about how you might be trying to help Jamie by remaining in her closet?

Jamie (speaking as her pants): *My job is to make sure Jamie stays a certain size so that she remains lovable. Getting rid of pants means she has gotten bigger.*

BodySelf: Can you tell us more about your worry? How did you come to believe outgrowing pants makes Jamie less lovable?

Jamie (speaking as her pants): *We learned from our family that outgrowing clothing, i.e. gaining weight, was bad. Smaller was always better. Getting bigger was dangerous; it led to criticism and hurtful comments.*

BodySelf: So, what do you think about the idea that maybe those beliefs might not "fit" Jamie anymore? Would you be willing to consider the idea that those worries and fears are from a different stage in Jamie's life? Have you noticed that now, Jamie feels loveable in many ways? Would you be open to considering that letting go of these beliefs might actually allow Jamie to feel even more loveable? The Jamie of today really wants to go shopping and find pants that feel good to her body and match her current style.

Jamie (speaking as pants): *That makes sense. I am willing to give it a try. I see that now I might not have to work so hard in the old ways to ensure that Jamie is loveable.*

Exercise 8.2 A Clothing Cure Mad Lib

Get curious about a piece of clothing you have held onto or that you try on intermittently. The ritual of trying it on might be an attempt to manage something from the past, present or future.

A piece of clothing I have held onto is my _____

If it fits, then that means that I am _____

When I wear _____ *and it fits, I feel* _____

Feeling this way is important to me because _____

If I can't fit into _____ *then it means* _____

_____

And I am _____

And I have to _____

Example:

A piece of clothing I have held onto is my black leather pants.

If they fit, then that means that I am still youthful and cool.

When I wear these pants *and they fit, I feel like* I still have style and am fun and full of life.

Feeling this way is important to me because as I get older, I worry about losing my youthful energy and the identity that goes with it.

If I can't fit into these pants *then it means* I am not youthful anymore.

And I am unsure what this next phase will be like, how I should dress and if people will still value me in the same way.

And I have to find something in between leather and linen that still feels like me!

Just like decoding your body image, you can decode clothing catastrophes and misfires and see what else might need to be heard and expressed.

Clothing Decoding Mini-Session: Grief Potato

BodySelf: Do you have a sense of where you might want to start today, what you are feeling curious about?

Molly: *I am feeling super vulnerable about my body, more than I have in months. This weekend I'm going to my cousin's wedding. I found a dress I felt really good about. It's flowy and comfortable and I really liked the way it looked on me when I bought it. But … I tried it on yesterday and again this morning and it looks awful.*

BodySelf: What's changed? What shift are you noticing in how you see yourself in the dress?

Molly: *It's sleeveless and while I love the pattern and how soft the fabric is, I suddenly feel so self-conscious and exposed. I feel like a potato with a dress on [laughter and tears].*

BodySelf: That is a big shift! Do you have any sense of what has happened in the weeks since buying the dress?

Molly: *I went home last weekend for my cousin's bridal shower and spent time with my whole family. You know how hard I have worked over the years to have firmer boundaries with my mom. Before I arrived, I felt so prepared and well-defended. Other than a few familiar mom-zingers, the weekend went surprisingly well. I am so used to feeling unsafe around her and focused on the best ways to protect myself. This past weekend, when my mom was actually more present and curious, I felt like, "What is happening? Can I let my guard down around her?" I have spent so many years building armor and appropriate expectations. Now I am kerfuffled.*

BodySelf: What are you noticing inside as you are sharing about the weekend?

Molly: *It's hard to hold both realities; I am so used to needing to be defended around her. It feels so new to have a positive interaction. I have worked so hard to release my expectations. Do I still need the armor I have built up all these years? I feel so vulnerable and confused.*

BodySelf: You are onto something important. What other feelings are you having after this weekend? I wonder if this vulnerability and confusion you are describing is impacting how you feel in your dress?

Molly: *I feel so confused and sad. You know about my mom's volatile moods and how lonely I felt growing up. There is a part of me that yearns to let my guard down and feel more connected to her and there is another part of me that is saying, "Protect yourself! Don't let her in again."*

BodySelf: It sounds like your mom showing up in a more approachable, engaged way actually brought up a lot for you. Does this feel right?

Molly: *Yes I am feeling confused. And ... I think I know what else I am feeling. Exposed. That is how I feel, EXPOSED!*

BodySelf: Well that is pretty interesting, because you started our conversation by talking about how "exposed" you felt in that dress!

Molly: *Woah, that is so true. I loved the dress and how I looked when I bought it ... but that totally shifted when I tried it on after my weekend with my mom. I think the question I really have is, "Can I expose myself to her or do I need to protect myself?" It's so hard to know whether I am safe enough to let my guard down. It makes so much sense that I feel vulnerable and exposed in a dress I plan to wear to the family wedding.*

> *"True belonging doesn't require you to change who you are; it requires you to be who you are."*
>
> Brené Brown

Our Clothes and "Fitting In"

We have heard endless stories that start with a piece of clothing not fitting and end with a fear about not "fitting in." Finding the right outfit often becomes code for, "Will I be accepted and feel like I belong?" Often, clothing holds the perceived power to tip the scale one way or another. When finding the right blazer feels like a life-changing decision, we can decode the actual stakes by asking the right questions to avoid a full-blown clothing catastrophe. In this section, you will learn to decode what parts of you are being expressed through your feelings about your clothing. Let's start with an example:

Client Spotlight: Perfect Cargo Pants

Sasha described being at T.J. Maxx at 10 p.m. the night before a college reunion hunting for the "perfect cargo pants." Sasha was in her early forties and single and deeply wanted to have a family of her own. She treasured her college friends and being with them was wonderful but also painful. They had all found partners and had children, which left her feeling like an outsider. While Sasha was on her flight to meet her friends, she did some writing about her late-night shopping odyssey and realized that what she had been looking for was the right "costume."

Casual, cool-looking cargo pants were what she imagined her friends wore in their day-to-day lives as moms, on the soccer sidelines or at school drop-off. Now she understood her late-night quest for those perfect cargo pants! "If I have the right pants, I will feel like I fit in that world and maybe they won't notice how different I am." Without knowing it, Sasha had directed her longing for a family and her desire to be less different than her friends into finding the right pants. Her unconscious hope was that the right pants could protect her from feelings of isolation and grief at the reunion.

It felt helpful to make these connections and when her plane landed, Sasha texted a good friend from work who was also single and let her know what she was grappling with. She also came up with a plan to share some of her feelings and fears about the weekend with the college friend she felt most comfortable with. Both of these actions allowed her to release her fixation on the pants by recognizing and resourcing the vulnerabilities she had hoped they would hide.

Sometimes not knowing what to wear is really about not knowing how to show up to a difficult conversation, circumstance or event.

Client Spotlight: What is My Heart Holding?

Maggie was in her late sixties and had a solid sense of her style. She felt even more grounded and confident with her wardrobe as she got older. However, when she was getting dressed for the funeral of her colleague's son, she was surprised to find herself staring at her entire wardrobe laid out on her bed and at a loss as to what to wear. Maggie had tried on almost every article of clothing she owned and still felt terrible about how she looked. She felt like she had somehow aged a decade and the force of gravity had doubled in the last 48 hours. Frustrated, she sat down on top of her layers of clothes, dropped her head in her hands and cried.

With four children of her own, imagining what her colleague must be going through gutted her. She realized at that moment that she did not know how to comfort her colleague in the face of such a devastating loss. Her feelings of vulnerability around her own children's health and safety pressed in on her. She had unconsciously hoped that finding the right outfit and looking strong would help manage the overwhelm in her heart. Once Maggie realized that no outfit could change the fact that she had no idea how to show up for this event, she was able to acknowledge her fear and helplessness and attend to those difficult emotions instead.

Exercise 8.3 "Fitting" In Our Clothes

Starting to notice and track your dialogue with your clothes is a great way to improve your relationship with your wardrobe. Pay particular attention to whenever you notice big feelings about getting dressed, regardless of if it is for a big event or everyday life.

What are the hardest places or events to get dressed for?

\
\

In what ways do you feel you fit in these settings? In what ways do you feel you don't?

\
\

How do you end up feeling towards your body when you are getting ready for these events?

\
\

If there are vulnerable feelings present, how could you support yourself and resource them?

\
\

Do you have something to wear that is "right enough" for these kinds of events?

\
\

When Our Clothes Talk Back

We invite you to consider how a piece of clothing *feels* to your insides rather than just how it *looks* on the outside. Clothing is a sensory experience, and you now know the importance of the relationship between sensations, body image and alignment. Sometimes we wear things because we think they look good even if they are uncomfortable. But, as we have learned, if our clothes make us feel uncomfortable by pinching, scratching or squishing, those sensations may make us feel worse as the day or night wears on. So we invite you to bring more awareness and curiosity to the sensory experience of your clothing.

Client Spotlight: Hard Pants

Gina was a dedicated teacher at an urban school. Like all teachers during the pandemic, she was asked to create a virtual classroom from home and spent hours on her computer teaching kids and coaching their parents. Despite this extremely stressful time, one aspect of teaching felt easier: getting dressed for work.

When her classroom reopened, Gina had to get ready for the first in-person teacher meeting. She tried on every pair of pants in her closet. Nothing looked right. Nothing was comfortable. So many feelings came up as she wondered, "Why is this so hard?" and realized that she hadn't gotten dressed for anything professional in person for over two years. Going back to being the "Miss Gina" from two years ago just felt wrong.

Gina had grown and changed in so many ways over the previous two years and she was committed to finding more ease and alignment wherever she could. Wearing "hard pants" (thank you pandemic for that endearing term) just didn't match up with how she wanted to dress as a first grade teacher anymore. She needed more comfortable pants. It was helpful for her to name the ways she wanted to adapt and align in this new chapter of her career, starting with her closet. Gina's wardrobe has since been updated to reflect her more flexible attitude and style.

Exercise 8.4 Clothing and Our Senses

I love wearing _____ **because** _____.

I like wearing _____ **because** _____.

I enjoy wearing _____ **because** _____.

Examples:

I love wearing my silk top **because** it's light and soft on my skin and covers my arms, which I feel self-conscious of.

I like wearing colorful sneakers **because** they never hurt my feet and make anything I am wearing a little more funky.

I enjoy wearing stretchy blazers **because** they make me feel confident, keep me warm and move with my body.

Style and Alignment

Now that you have started to decode your clothing, let's use these new insights to help you find more alignment and resonance through fashion and style, or as Rachel Zoe describes, "say who you are without having to speak." Let's start by distinguishing style from fashion. *Fashion* is a reflection of current trends—the length of our skirt, the cut of our jeans, wearing neutrals or vivid hues. *Style* is about expressing our individuality through combinations of color, design, fabric, texture and overall vibe. Style is the act of showcasing identity and uniqueness through clothing and accessories. Playing with personal style can be an opportunity to explore aspects of ourselves and evolve as we do.

Maybe you love to read about the newest trends from "Fashion Week" and recreate them in your own way, or maybe you prefer to wear your favorite T-shirt in four different colors. Perhaps you seek out signature pieces from well-known designers or shop from companies that prioritize sustainability. You might love to thrift to find the perfect jumpsuit or leather jacket. While there is often a frivolity associated with investing in clothing, we believe it can be a profoundly valuable playground for building new skills and connecting to ourselves.

"The most controversial act I have ever committed in my life is being true to myself."

Sherenté

Client Spotlight: Counter-cultural Evolution

Natalie grew up in a close and connected Jewish family, with a strong currency around being together and sharing the same interests. Vacations and holidays were always spent together, and there were often party themes, activities and dress codes that everyone was expected to partake in. In Natalie's early life, this family culture felt fun and gave her a sense of belonging, but as she moved into adolescence and noticed the ways that she felt different, she didn't know how to express her individuality without jeopardizing family connection. Over time, it became increasingly clear that she was more drawn to vintage than high fashion, backpacking instead of the beach and dating women rather than men. This made it challenging for her to feel aligned with herself and comply with the dress code for family events.

It was a difficult process for Natalie to discover what resonated for her and how to express this within her family. It took years, but ultimately she found the courage to wear a T-shirt and board shorts on their beach vacations and even suggested some alternative family events like hiking and football games where fashion wasn't the headline.

One definition of alignment is "to be in agreement or alliance with ourselves." Natalie's story demonstrates how playing with our clothing helps us clarify what feels "in agreement with ourselves." Figuring out how we want to express ourselves through clothing that feels right to us and navigating the challenges it may pose in our relationships, can become a process of becoming more aligned with our unique "brand."

> *"There is something really magical about a person getting dressed and being able to convey: This is the mood I am in, this is how I want to be seen. To me, that's art."*
>
> Na Kim

Client Spotlight: The Heels that Changed My Life

Kate grew up in a small rural town where she never felt like she fit in with her peers. She was interested in the arts, travel and education, while most of her peers were playing school sports or video games. In her community, being different was strongly discouraged, so Kate stuck to the prescribed look of her peers (jeans, sweatshirts, hightops) and kept her dreams of a more adventurous life to herself.

The world opened up to Kate when she received a scholarship to a liberal arts college in a big city. She challenged her rural roots with bright red lipstick and pleather pants and even got a tattoo. But it took six months of walking past the pole dancing studio on her commute to her internship to have the courage to sign up for a class.

She had never loved anything more: the physicality (she had loved gymnastics as a kid), the techno music … and then there were the heels. Her body just kept saying "Yes! When I wear these crazy high sparkly heels, I feel strong and gorgeous and sexy!" In her apartment, she left her sparkly red shoes on display on a shelf because looking at them felt like a wink to herself.

The clothing attached to a beloved activity can come to represent the parts of us that come alive through that endeavor. It could be your first rugby team jersey, the apron your grandmother gave you when the two of you baked together or the necklace you wore at your first keynote speech. These meaningful pieces represent important parts of ourselves.

"Weirdos. Will. Slay. Because not fitting in to any one community is a super power. But only if you fit into yourself first."

Sebane Selassie

Our Closet from the Inside Out

By the time we are old enough to buy our own clothes, we have taken in so many messages about how we should look that getting dressed often becomes another way to "get it right." If you have been struggling with body image, chances are you have been trying to contort your "puzzle piece." We see getting dressed as an opportunity to align more with our own puzzle piece. Standing in front of our closet can be a cue to ask, "How am I feeling today, and what clothes would best support me?" Rather than trying to fit into clothes, clothing gets to fit onto us and be what we need it to be: comfort, expression, alignment, protection and support.

Getting dressed can be a chance for you to experiment with a more authentic version of yourself. This can be an opportunity to practice noticing when you are connected to yourself and getting curious when you aren't.

Getting Dressed Daily Practice: The BodySelf Way

To feel more alignment and authenticity in our second skin, ask these questions as you get dressed.

- What are three words to describe how I feel/want to feel today?
- What wants to be expressed?
- What needs to be nurtured?
- What would feel good to my skin? Something soft? Something warm?
- What would feel good to my other senses?
- Do I want something colorful, loud, edgy, neutral, professional?

Exercise 8.5 Aligning With Our Closet

When we give our closet our attention, energy and creativity for the sake of greater alignment, we set ourselves up to be able to use clothing as a love language. Let's get curious about when you feel confident, relaxed or in some way aligned with yourself. What are the things you do that bring you that sense of alignment AND are there certain pieces of clothing that support feeling connected to yourself?

When do you feel the most aligned and like YOU? List three answers:

1. _____

2. _____

3. _____

Example:

When do you feel the most like YOU? List three answers:

1 Before I go out for the evening, when I am getting ready, listening to my favorite music and dancing alone.

2 When I am with people I love, when I feel at ease with myself and am feeling most truly ME.

3 The moment I get off a plane in a place I have never been before.

Which pieces of clothing help you feel connected to yourself? List three answers:

1. _____

2. _____

3. _____

Example:

Which pieces of clothing help you feel connected to yourself? List three answers:

1 My super soft flannel pajamas.

2 My matchy-matchy Lycra bike "kit."

3 My vibrant floral kimono and ripped jeans.

Here are some questions to help you identify if the items of clothing you currently have are keepers or not.

Closet Inventory

You can use the following questions to help you bring more presence and alignment to your relationship with the clothes you own.

How does this piece of clothing make me feel?

_____

_____

Is it a "should" or a "want" piece of clothing?

_____

_____

What sensations do I notice in my body when I look at it?

_____

_____

What sensations do I notice in my body when I have it on?

_____

_____

What do I feel when I think about keeping it or letting it go?

_____

_____

Suggested clearing actions:

- Items that are not comfortable, either because of how they feel on our bodies or that they don't feel aligned with our style.
- Clothes that have "shoulds" attached to them and don't make us feel good (i.e. everyone "should" have a _____).
- Clothes that we are holding onto for reasons other than alignment, i.e. they were on sale, they were expensive, we are hoping to fit into them someday in the future.

- You have options after removing them from your closet: you can donate them, you can see if any friends want them or you can put them in storage and revisit in three months if it is hard to let them go.

Suggested cultivating actions:

- Get clear about what colors you love to wear.
- Figure out what clothing fit, shape, patterns and styles you feel good in or are drawn to.
- Create a Pinterest or mood board with styles that inspire you and that you might want to explore.
- Find someone to help you investigate an aligned closet: a friend or a consultant, especially if this process feels isolating and/or hard.
- Cultivate an open, ongoing conversation with your closet and your clothes—it's an ongoing practice.
- Are there other actions that come to mind?

Body Image Super Bowls: High-Stakes Events

We couldn't write a section about body image and clothing and not address high-stakes events such as weddings, reunions and graduations. Weddings are always at the top of the list because so many people grapple with the complicated emotions that are activated around a wedding, whether you are the bride, the best man, a distant cousin or a friend at the singles table. Being a bride or groom comes with an extremely high level of pressure, particularly surrounding how one "should" look and feel on their big day. We are socialized to assume that the bride and groom will look their best *and* those around them will too. And if we aren't basking in the wedding blueprint feelings of excitement and bliss, we can feel like there is something wrong with us. What a set-up for a BBIM! We often hear things like: "The expectations feel huge," "I felt too much," "My feelings were so big." It can be really helpful to remind ourselves that the strong feelings we have on these big days might very well trickle into how we are feeling in our body and our clothing.

Here are a few examples of how the emotions around *high-stakes events* can get expressed either through a BBIM or a clothing kerfuffle and are opportunities for BodySelf reframes:

Our Body Image says: This is my fifth wedding this spring—I have worn the same dress to every single one and I am so sick of it! When I put it on, I feel old and tired.

Our BodySelf says: *This is my fifth wedding this spring and I am dating up a storm, but can't find the right partner. I am so tired from the energy it takes to show up for my friends and try to find my person.*

Our Body Image says: I can't find anything to wear to my father's wedding. I haven't seen him in a decade and I can't seem to find a dress that feels right. Everything makes me feel like I'm trying too hard.

Our BodySelf says: *I have been invited to attend the wedding of my estranged father and nothing feels like the right thing to wear. Who sells dresses for shitty dad weddings? Everything I put on feels fake and forced. Maybe that's because that's how this whole experience makes me feel.*

Our Body Image says: I am going away for the weekend with my new boyfriend to his high school reunion. I have gone shopping four times and everything I try on looks awful. I keep buying things and then returning them.

Our BodySelf says: *I am going away for the weekend with my new boyfriend to his high school reunion. I imagine I will be the only woman of color there given that he went to a small Catholic school in rural Pennsylvania. I worry I am going to stand out no matter what I wear and it makes so much sense that I feel like I can't get my outfit right.*

Our Body Image says: I cannot figure out what to wear to my big work event next weekend. I have borrowed clothes from my sisters and friends and gone through everything in my closet and I just can't find anything that looks even passable.

Our BodySelf says: *I am headed to a big work training for all the people at my company who got promoted. The invitations said the dress code is "resort chic." I have no idea what that means. I don't like small talk, drinking gives me migraines and I fear I'll be uncomfortable the whole time. I'm worried that I wont be able to find anyone I genuinely want to connect with.*

Client Spotlight: A BodySelf Bride

Liv had grown up with two parents who were loving and well-intentioned but quite body-obsessed. From a young age, Liv felt highly self-conscious of her size and she worked hard to address the ways her parents' values had impacted her. When she and her girlfriend got engaged, she was thrilled but also worried about the sharp focus on appearance and perfection that weddings activate. She committed herself to making the wedding planning experience as aligned and intentional as possible.

Liv had always felt self-conscious of her fingers and feared the ring shopping process was going to be uncomfortable at best. Liv and her fiancée chose a jeweler who was recommended for her interpersonal skills and creativity. Their experience was unexpectedly fun and Liv surprised herself when she found a ring she loved. Liv had even greater anxiety about dress shopping but with the ring experience under her belt, she had a blueprint for how she wanted to feel in the process.

Liv sought out a bridal shop she heard was "queer friendly" because she was unsure if she wanted to wear a dress or a suit. While the boutique was lovely, Liv knew this wasn't her place when the saleswoman said to her, "That dress is so flattering on you." "Flattering" is a word Liv had heard endlessly growing up and was code for "that makes you look thin." Liv remembered how the jeweler made her feel and how much curiosity she held for Liv's process in choosing the ring. "If I focus on being skinny (i.e what is "flattering"), I can't figure out what I love. I want to pay attention to how the dress or suit feels to *me*!" She found another boutique and ultimately a suit she adored.

There is no recipe for ease and self-love on these profoundly important days in our lives but as Liv demonstrated, there are many ways to notice our inner messages and longings and course-correct when we need to.

Exercise 8.6 Big Event Survival Kit

Attending big events may rattle some of your relational mirrors and kick up some BBIMs for sure. It can be valuable to think about the event in three phases to minimize the negative impact on your body image.

Phase 1: Preparing for the event:

What is the event or situation coming up?

_____

_____

Who do you feel like you are dressing for?

_____

_____

What's the wish or fantasy? What do you want them to "see" and why?

_____

_____

How do you want to feel in your body?

_____

_____

*How do you anticipate your body image might try to step in during the event
and how might your respond?*

_____

_____

Who or what might help you feel more connected to yourself or supported?

_____

_____

*Is there anything you can imagine needing after the event that you could put
into place now?*

_____

_____

Phase 2: Being at the event:

*If you had a note in the palm of your hand that you could use for reassurance
during the event, what would it say to you?*

_____

_____

If you had someone by your side during the event, who would it be and why?

_____

_____

Phase 3: Resourcing after the event:

*Can you congratulate yourself for the ways you navigated the event that felt
good to you?*

_____

_____

What did you enjoy/not enjoy about the event?

_____

_____

What is your body image saying?

_____

_____

How can you resource yourself given all of this?

_____

_____

Super Bowl Recap

- Big events bring up big feelings and emotions far beyond the question of what to wear.
- We often try to manage these feelings by focusing on how we look at the event.
- The previously mentioned big emotions can get redirected into feelings towards our body and what we are wearing.
- We can prepare for these events to minimize their negative impact and celebrate and resource ourselves when we make it to the other side.

Bless the colors, textures and styles that light you up.

*May this collection of garments become
an alignment playground.*

*May you use your clothes each day to get closer to what
feels aligned with you—Bless your Yes's and No's.*

*May the BBIMs and bad hair days bring you opportunities to
flex your new muscles.*

May the excellent outfits encourage your growing self-trust.

Your closet is now in service of you and your BodySelf.

9 | The Art of Resourcing Ourselves

"Your body is both a lens of perception and an instrument of action."

Amanda Blake

Now that we are off the fix-it or hate-it treadmill and we know more about what our body is communicating, how do we figure out what it needs and how to support ourselves, aka "resource ourselves?" To answer this question, we will be sharing skills and practices.

What is Resourcing?

Our negative body image rotary patterns have been trying to help us out through habitual responses that temporarily distract us from our needs or emotional upset. In the past, our body image stepped in as strongly as it did because we didn't have what we needed to resource ourselves. So while it was creative and adaptive for our body image to try and help us, it kept us from accessing what we really needed. Our negative body image said: "*Hating and fixing* your body will make this better." Resourcing says: "Let's get you *what you need* right now to make this better." It brings the process full circle by actually attending to the longings and needs body image could only temporarily distract you from.

We want to help you learn to listen and respond to your inner cues. Do we need to tell someone they have hurt us, set a limit in response to their behavior, ask for help or reward ourselves? Do we simply need to attend to our feelings? Clarifying what we need may take some time. When we have been listening to our body negativity shout out automatic solutions for so long, it will take practice to learn to listen to our body's more authentic voice. This is especially tricky because, as we have said, most of us haven't been socialized to be connected to our bodies. In fact, many, if not most environments tacitly discourage it. We live in a culture that encourages and rewards us for abandoning our bodies for success. In fact, most work cultures praise us for going above and beyond. Even high-level athletes who represent the peak of health and embodiment are trained to override their bodies' cues around fatigue and discomfort. For most of us, the pace of life exceeds what is ideal and listening to our bodies is a more subtle and less celebrated skill.

Resourcing Skill: Resonance

In her famous poem, "Wild Geese," poet Mary Oliver invites us to "let the soft animal of your body love what it loves," to allow ourselves to like what we like, with the deep instincts of an animal who has not been trained to overthink or "should." Learning to let our body "love what it loves" is an ongoing practice of alignment: listening and experimenting. It means getting clear about what we feel, what we need and want, and then resourcing ourselves accordingly. Knowing how to figure out what aligns with us is vital to the process of resourcing ourselves well.

Our body is our primary tool when it comes to interpreting our response to our environments. Negative body image training has repeatedly told us that our body is wrong and it needs to be fixed. To counteract this training, practice listening to how your body responds to what it likes and dislikes. In doing this, we are replacing years of training of being in disagreement with how our body looks and feels, with learning what our body agrees with. Alignment is learning the language of your body's yes's and we practice this by listening for resonance.

If awareness and sensation had a baby, it would be resonance. Resonance is the feeling we get when our body is in agreement with external stimuli; it's the gateway to finding more alignment in our lives. How does your body feel inside when something feels "right" to you? It could be "chills" up and down your arms, an airy lightness in your stomach or a sense of anchoring along your spine.

Client Spotlight: On the Move

Andrea was a financial analyst and a master's level cross-country skier. Having competed on elite teams for over a decade, she missed the hours of outdoor training and camaraderie of skiing with others. She had a muscular build and a bit of a tan from training outside. All her friends and work colleagues made direct and indirect comments about how "healthy" she was, assuming that she was comfortable and confident in her body.

But in reality, Andrea was only "embodied" when she was training or racing, finding the correct placement of her poles and angle of her skis relative to the terrain. She was aware of how she was carrying her head and the position of her torso. She knew the impact of micro adjustments to her posture and effort levels. But when she wasn't moving, Andrea had a hard time feeling present in her body. She was restless and wiggly in her skin.

Andrea started to address this ever-present discomfort with a sports psychologist and realized that all the challenges in her home life as a kid, the ones that her competitive skiing career took her away from, were still within her. The focus and endorphins of exercise and the anxiety of the next race or work deadline kept her temporarily distracted over and over again. Andrea was exquisitely embodied on the race course, and had an entirely different relationship with her body when she was at rest. With support, Andrea was able to meet and transform her pain for the first time, allowing her to find a new way of relating to herself and her body.

Resourcing Skill: Alignment

Sentences that start with "I just knew ..." capture alignment. It's that sense of congruence inside us, that something feels in sync with our being. Ever have an outdated shirt or pair of shoes you just love and, even though they aren't exactly the latest trend, you get more compliments on them than anything else you own? Or that feeling when a book, song or show feels like it was written or made for you? It's that resonance inside us when we finally find the right paint color for our bedroom when our sample wall looks like a patchwork quilt. It's knowing which friend to call when we are struggling. Alignment is when the natural puzzle piece that lives inside our body and a puzzle piece outside of us ... click together easily.

While much of our lives may have involved vilifying the body and trying to change it, our body can be a powerful antenna for alignment. For most of us, finding alignment wasn't something we were taught to recognize or cultivate. It takes practice to become more connected to our bodies, to receive its information and to listen for resonance.

Exercise 9.1 Connecting to Your Alignment

Resonance is learning the language of your body's yes's. Let's practice:

What art, music, book or _____ feels like it was created for you? How do you know that?

_____

_____

Who are the people you feel drawn to (celebrities, authors, public figures)? How do you know that?

_____

_____

How do you know more generally when something resonates for you? What sensations accompany, "this feels right?"

_____

_____

Think of the last time, place or experience felt like a "Yes" in your body. What sensations told you it was a "Yes?"

_____

_____

Is there anything that feels challenging about listening to your body or being more in tune with it?

_____

_____

Once you get more familiar with what your inner resonance feels like, you can build more trust in your body's version of "Yes!" and use this information to build more alignment in your life.

- **Negative Body Image** says, "Something is wrong with you (and your body) and you need to change it."
- **Alignment** says, "There is nothing wrong with you or your body. I want to know, what are you and your body feeling, needing, longing for? What does the 'soft animal of your body' love?"

> *"To be embodied means that we let the intelligence of our body-sensations, energies and intuition inform and guide our life."*
>
> Tami Simon

We all have aspects of our life where we don't have a lot of flexibility or choice. We invite you to start to look for small opportunities to choose what feels more aligned. Here are some examples:

- Skipping the last module of a training or leaving the conference early when we are exhausted.
- Seeking out help on a project that is overwhelming or where we lack expertise.
- Finding mentors in areas of our life where we are wanting to grow.
- Reaching out to a friend when we are struggling when usually we tough it out alone.
- Organizing a walk or hike with friends when we are wishing and longing for time in open spaces.
- Seeking specialists or services in our community to help with an aging parent or a child who might need more support rather than bearing the full responsibility.

Boundaries: "No's" Can Reveal Deeper "Yes's"

A big part of practicing alignment is realizing what *doesn't* feel right to you, where there *isn't* resonance. This concept may seem counterintuitive because you may think of alignment as things you want to say "yes" to, things that you want more of in your life. Often boundaries are seen as a rejection. Author William Urich says that there is no such thing as a "no" when it comes to setting boundaries, simply a deeper yes. If you say "no" to a dinner party, you are saying "yes" to staying home. If you say "no" to buying something you really liked, you are saying "yes" to using that money in a different way. If you say "no" to leading a project at work, you are saying "yes" to having time and energy for what is already on your plate. So getting clear on your "no's" and learning how to communicate them is a big part of building alignment in your life.

Boundaries are an integral part of the transformation from living a life in service of shapeshifting to living in greater alignment with your BodySelf. To do this, we will inevitably practice getting clearer on our deeper yes's. Though boundaries ultimately preserve our wellbeing, we often feel uneasy when saying "no." Like all muscles, setting boundaries is strengthened by repetition, and the shaky feeling we may get when we are saying "no" tells you that this is something that matters. Over time, you will develop more courage and confidence and the shakiness will dissipate. So let's talk about what to expect when you start to build more boundaries and how to practice them.

- Start by identifying what does *not* feel aligned: *Not* this pair of pants, *not* this way of spending time, *not* this person who treats me poorly. In the beginning, noticing what is a "not this" as you go through your day may be easier than recognizing what feels aligned.

- Be patient. In practicing these new boundaries, it can be helpful to take the pressure off of making any actual changes in behavior, and just allow yourself to register what feels like a "not this."

- Identify what is most important to you right now. To get clear on your yes's, it can be helpful to think through what yes's you want to protect? What are your top five to eight values? For example: time with friends, being in nature, getting enough sleep, loyalty, honesty. My top values are:

_____

_____

_____

_____

When we start to set boundaries, we don't have to suddenly stop talking to people or quit our job. There are so many small moments in which to practice. Setting a boundary can be realizing on page 55 of the new book we are reading that although we love this author, we are not loving her latest novel and putting it down. Or it's deciding to go for a walk instead of a run because it feels better to our body. It can be ordering takeout because we are exhausted or because it just makes us happy.

Client Spotlight: From Counting Calories to Counting Yes's

Priti was an executive director in a large accounting firm. She had four children, one of whom had ADHD and needed a lot of her attention to manage his academics. Her husband recently left his job to start his own company, but so far that wasn't going very well, and she was feeling the pressure of being the sole breadwinner. Having recently gone through menopause, she noticed that she was "carrying her weight differently," and had less energy and focus for the considerable amount on her plate. Though she hadn't struggled much with negative body image since before her children were born, Priti found herself counting calories and obsessing over what foods increase metabolism. She felt her schedule and responsibilities had "shoved her out of her body" as she had no time to attend to it. She could barely get her hair cut let alone exercise or sleep in on the weekends like she used to.

Priti enlisted the help of a nutritionist, who helped her see that her current diet focus was taking up too much space in her head and diminishing her energy levels. Through these conversations, Priti discovered that food was only a part of the picture, and what she was really craving was more room in her life to attend to her body and its changing needs. Together, she and the nutritionist came up with both lifestyle and food-related strategies to respond to what body image was trying to help her with. She became clear on her yes's and started to slowly create more boundaries with her time and outsource some of her work at home and in the office.

Resourcing is bringing people, places, activities or objects to ourselves for the purpose of giving ourselves what we actually need.

Resourcing Practice: Self-care

"Self-care" is a term that gets a lot of airtime and can mean something different to each of us. Author Lalah Delia calls self-care "a love language to the body." Lifestyle guru Tim Ferris defines it as, "building and recharging one's energetic reservoir." Self-care is an exercise in listening to our body and running experiments to discover what nourishes us. We get to create our own love language and fill our own reservoir.

Self-care can feel loaded; some have been taught that it is indulgent or selfish, others don't feel clear about what would feel good or fear they won't do it "right." And there are so many messages and platforms that preach the perfect path to bliss. We might have no idea what feels good to us because we have never been encouraged to ask ourselves or given ourselves permission to explore self-care. It might actually feel like trying to find a location without a map or an address. The good news is our body holds great wisdom, and we can start exploring possibilities and listening to what our body has to say in response. Self-care is deeply personal and we give you a giant permission slip to trust that it is OK to discover your unique recipe for self-care.

> *"Self-care is choosing a life that feels good over one that looks good."*
>
> Shenikka Moore-Clarke

Why is Self-care Important to The BodySelf?

It might sound bananas, but focusing on, fixing or changing our body might have felt like a form of self-care. It may have offered a private and accessible way to tend to ourselves and our hurts when we didn't have other tools to handle or process overwhelming aspects of our lives. The trouble is, it was probably based on a "should" rather than something we actually wanted. Using "should" language can feel protective because it might keep our identities intact.

- I "should" work through lunch to get this done, but I really want to go and get a yummy lunch and a change of scenery.
- I just got back from a big trip and I'm exhausted. I "should" unpack and go to the gym, but actually I really want a nap.
- I "should" get that person a really expensive wedding present because they have fancy taste even though I am on a tight budget.
- I "should" wear heels to this event even though I really want to wear my stylish sneakers. They are so much more comfortable, funky and more me.

What is important about moving from "should" to "want" anyway? Isn't life full of things we should do? Yes and Yes. We don't need to ignore our "shoulds"—there are lots of things that we need to tend to in our lives and "shoulds" get the job done. *AND* we invite you to notice the language you use as you make choices during your day, as it might offer more information about what your body actually needs. Bring awareness to when you are "shoulding yourself" and then ask, "Does this feel right? Is this really what I want?" For example, "I should make a meal for my friend who is sick *and* I want to just order her take-out." "I should get this report in by tonight *and* I haven't spent time with my daughter lately. I want to snuggle and read with her and finish the report in the morning." Simply inviting that little word *AND* into your life can help you allow room for *want* to get some airtime. Most of us have been socialized to "should" so much that we don't even realize we might be overriding our body cues and that we have a different choice. Self-care is an opportunity for our body to move from "should" to "want".

> *"I want to be concerned about what I want,*
> *not whether I am wanted."*
>
> Glennon Doyle

Self-care is how we practice valuing ourselves. It transitions us away from seeing our value in terms of units of productivity, measures of attractiveness or what others want from or for us. When we lose connection to ourselves, self-care is a direct portal back to connection. If you have spent your life trying to shapeshift yourself rather than connect to yourself, this may take some time.

How Do you Practice Self-care?

Let's figure out what self-care looks like for you. Yes, the research shows that seven to eight hours of sleep, hydration and eating fruits and vegetables are all great forms of self-care. And some people need to start there. But there are many other options, and self-care isn't one-size-fits-all. Respect your own heart's desires. While one person might feel recharged by an interval workout on a track, another might prefer a yoga class and a third might prefer a slow walk in the woods. If you long for the walk in the woods option and you choose the track interval workout to check the "self-care box," it won't recharge you as much.

We invite you to practice what Behida Dolića calls a "little gesture of the soul." It could be getting a pedicure, sitting in the park for lunch, putting on fake eyelashes or making time for pickup basketball on Friday nights. So say yes to buying that little plant you love at the grocery store, making sure you make time to watch a favorite show, reading that hardcover book, meeting the dogs at the dog park ... all of it is self-care. The next time you do something for yourself, notice how it FEELS to look at your purple manicured toes or to have your favorite beer or dessert at the end of a crappy day. Observe what happens in your body, what shifts, expands or dissipates. Run experiments and observe the results. That is how we start learning what our system needs.

Exercise 9.2 Self-care Inventory

What are some current ways you take care of yourself that are really working for you?

_____

_____

What are your self-care non-negotiable practices or rituals?

_____

_____

What are some current ways you take care of yourself that are no longer resonant?

_____

_____

*What are ways others engage in self-care that appeal to you? Are there some
that you are drawn to but haven't yet given yourself permission to try?*

How would you like to engage in self-care a year from now?

What If Self-care Feels Hard?

One of our favorite yoga teachers always says "Savasana," where you simply lie
on your mat in stillness, is the hardest yoga pose there is, much more challenging
than some fancy headstand or balancing pose. Your striving and achievement
("should") oriented parts will likely push back when you start exploring self-care.
They may feel threatened by *receiving instead of efforting.* Notice these parts, let
them know that you hear them and thank them for all the ways they help you
move through the world. Then ask them if they are willing to step back a bit so you
can run some experiments to discover how self-care impacts *you* and *your unique*
body. Your pushing and driving energy may still feel like it needs to show up *and*
we encourage you to run self-care experiments anyway, to remember you have
choices and a body that can help you deeply care for yourself.

> *"Self-care is how you take your power back."*
>
> Lalah Delia

Resourcing Practice: Cultivating Your Dream Team

Learning to give ourselves resources that are aligned with our wants and
needs—externally and internally—is a primary aim of the BodySelf process. Up
until now, most of your retraining has been invisible and happening on the inside.
This step is where it all meets the world. To come into a new way of moving
through life with a better relationship with our body image, we need to do it in
relationship with others. There are many ways to resource ourselves relationally;
one of the best ways is to build our support team.

Through resourcing, we practice noticing not only what feeds us but also which
choices feel the most supportive. We experiment with allowing our needs and
vulnerabilities to be seen and asking others for help. In the beginning, it might
feel indulgent to let anyone help us, especially when we have been overriding our

needs for so long. There is no template when it comes to resourcing. There is just inviting more alignment and people alongside us to help. Who we choose to have on our team of supporters will be influenced by many factors. We will also likely have different options depending on our stage of life. Living in alignment is not the absence of struggle, rather it is learning how to take care of ourselves as we go through the inevitable challenges of life.

So who the heck do you put on a BodySelf Dream Team? There is no right answer. We'll just offer a few ideas:

- Friends
- Movement community: a running club, yoga, dance, martial arts class you enjoy, a trainer or walking buddy
- Communities built around a neighborhood, spiritual orientation, activism, profession or hobby including both mentors and peers
- Psychotherapist, life or executive coach or psychiatrist
- Bodyworkers: massage therapist, acupuncturist, chiropractor or practitioner of other somatic therapies
- Physician, nurse practitioner and/or physical therapist

Over time, our bodies, needs, vulnerabilities and strengths shift and how we resource ourselves evolves. Resourcing asks us to continue to be curious and to listen to our bodies and our needs as they change.

Exercise 9.3 Dream Team Check-in

Let's take stock of your current roster. Who is currently on your dream team?

_____ *because they support me by:*

_____

_____

_____ *because they support me by:*

_____

_____

_____ *because they support me by:*

_____

_____

Who would you like to add to your dream team?

I need more support in the area of:

_____

_____

One action step I could take to get this support is:

_____

_____

I need more guidance with:

_____

_____

One action step I could take to get this support:

_____

_____

I need more aliveness in the area of:

_____

_____

One action step I could take to get more support:

_____

_____

"The world needs (people) who stop asking for permission from the principal. Permission to live their lives as they deeply know they often should. I think we still look to authority figures for validation, recognition, permission."

Elizabeth Gilbert

Resourcing Practice: Permission Slips

As is evident from the client spotlights in this book, as well as thousands of other anecdotal data points, most people find it hard to receive even a compliment. Many have been conditioned to get their needs met by meeting other people's needs, or making themselves more appealing, i.e. shapeshifting. Shapeshifting is a very indirect route to receiving and one that relies on the other person's needs and our effort. This subject could be a book in itself, but what is most important to know is that receiving may be a new muscle that requires practice. And first, you may only be able to receive small amounts of what feels good. It can be a stretch to go from people-pleasing to suddenly resourcing yourself well in all areas of your life, as it would be to go from having never run a race to being marathon-ready overnight. Resourcing takes practice and intentionality. And don't be surprised if it is uncomfortable at first. A great way to practice is to hand yourself small permission slips: permission to say no to little things, permission to take in a tiny bit of that compliment, permission to splurge on something you like with your time or your money, permission to try new experiences outside of your receiving comfort zone.

Exercise 9.4 Write Yourself a Permission Slip

Take a moment to think of all that you have read so far in this chapter.

What has become more clear to you after reading this chapter?

_____

_____

What has become more clear about what you allow yourself?

_____

_____

What has become more clear about what you want?

_____

_____

Can you imagine giving yourself something that you want or want more of in your life?

_____

_____

What fear or hesitation arises?

_____

_____

Can you write yourself a permission slip despite that resistance to go for that thing you want?

_____

_____

> *"You yourself, as much as anybody in the entire universe, deserve your love and affection."*
>
> Buddha

🌿 **PERMISSION SLIP** 🌿

I, _____ *grant myself permission*

to _____

I will rely on _____ *as an*

accountability partner, and I will turn to

_____ *for support. I am*

practicing resourcing myself.

Signed: _____ *Date:* _____

🌿 🌿 🌿 🌿 🌿 🌿 🌿

*The world is rich in offering and
full of sensory experiences.*

*Ease, nourishment, beauty and
connection are your birthright.*

*You are not here simply to bless,
but to allow yourself to be blessed.*

*One of the most lovely things you can do
is to deeply receive and to enjoy yourself.*

10 | The BodySelf Way

"I don't want to waste any of my life not being who I am."

Jonathan Van Ness

The BodySelf goal has never been to help you achieve perfect body image but to practice coming back to yourself. We are constantly transforming, both internally and externally, and our bodies are in a continual state of flux. Investing time in nurturing our relationship with our body image allows us to reconnect with ourselves, again and again, throughout life's changes. Body image work isn't linear; it is more like the seasons, forever evolving and returning.

Your Body Image Isn't Meant to "Arrive"

We all have times when we feel more freedom from negative body image and times when we will need to come back to the BodySelf practices. Thankfully, when we find ourselves in what feels like an epic BBIM, we can investigate what is causing us to feel the desire to change ourselves and identify ways to resource our true needs. You absolutely will still have negative body image thoughts in the future, but now you have choices in how you respond.

So what does a BodySelf practice really look like and how do you know you are doing it right? There is no *right* way; there is a practice of creating more space so that you can hear what your body image is communicating. Your BodySelf practice will ultimately be made up of:

- Tools from this book: mindful awareness, curiosity, compassion, decoding, self-care, alignment and resourcing
- Your intuition and creativity
- Your experiments and practice

Putting It All Together

Here is what it looks like to bring the full BodySelf approach and everything you have learned in the previous chapters to the Rotary experience:

1 You experience overwhelming feelings.

2 Your big feelings, thoughts and sensations get redirected towards your body, aka a BBIM.

3 ~~You decide to fix your body and create a plan.~~

4 ~~You get focused on the action (diet, exercise, etc.) and distracted from the overwhelming feelings.~~

5 ~~The emotions that are fueling bad body image don't get addressed and continue to drive a body fix.~~

6 ~~A pattern for fixing the body gets laid down and is likely to repeat.~~

Now let's bring in the BodySelf approach:

7 Use **mindful awareness** to recognize you are in a pattern. Remember you can BodySelf this moment.

8 Get **curious**. Ask yourself, what might be **triggering** me? Why is my **body image so loud** right now?

9 Bring **compassion**. Recognize that these patterns are driven by emotional pain and you have the ability to support yourself.

10 Turn your body image inside out and **decode**.

11 What are three possible options for how you could **resource** yourself? Which of those feels the most aligned?

Exciting Your Rotary

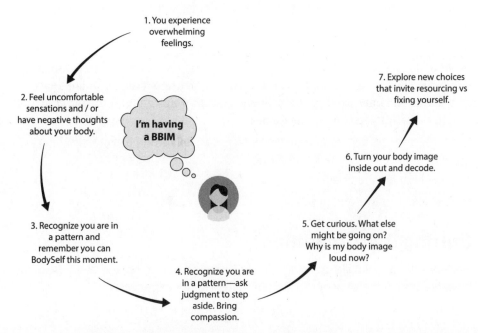

1. You experience overwhelming feelings.

2. Feel uncomfortable sensations and / or have negative thoughts about your body.

I'm having a BBIM

3. Recognize you are in a pattern and remember you can BodySelf this moment.

4. Recognize you are in a pattern—ask judgment to step aside. Bring compassion.

5. Get curious. What else might be going on? Why is my body image loud now?

6. Turn your body image inside out and decode.

7. Explore new choices that invite resourcing vs fixing yourself.

Exercise 10.1 The BodySelf Rotary

It's time to flex your BodySelf muscles and practice all the skills you have learned. Let's get back to that BBIM from Chapter 4 and complete the journey off your rotary:

1 You experience overwhelming feelings.

2 Your big feelings, thoughts and sensations get directed towards your body, aka a BBIM.

3 You decide to fix your body and create a plan.

4 Use *mindful awareness* to recognize you are in a pattern. Remember you can BodySelf this moment.

5 Get *curious*. Ask yourself, what might be *triggering* me? Why is my *body image so loud* right now?

6 Bring *compassion*. Recognize that these patterns are driven by emotional discomfort and you have the ability to support yourself.

7 **Decode:** Turn your body image inside out—What are the words I am using to describe my uncomfortable body part, and how might this relate to my current situation?

_____

_____

_____

Decoding example:

The words I use to describe my uncomfortable belly are **full, big and like a thousand butterflies.** The way I think these words relate to my current life situation is that this is a **big** decision and I feel **full** of intense feelings and emotions about it. And I often feel **butterflies** when I am nervous or excited about something and I do feel both of those feelings. And, when I think about it, butterflies also represent transformation and buying a house is a huge, long-awaited change in my life.

8 **Resource:** What are three possible options for how you could resource yourself? Which of those feels the most aligned?

_____

_____

_____

Resourcing Example:

Since I am understandably having so many big feelings about this major life decision, how can I take care of these big feelings right now? I could talk to my friend Maya because she just bought a house and probably had some big feelings herself. I could go for a walk outside because that always helps me think more clearly and feel calmer. I could go to Target and buy something for the new house so I can channel some of this nervous energy. I think I might do all three!

New Terrain

Congratulations! This is an entirely different way of responding to your negative body image. If you have made it this far, you are open, curious, dedicated and well on your way to practicing a new way of being in relationship with your body. And we want to honor that the reward for such bravery is not only the myriad of possibilities that come with a more connected relationship with your body, but likely some discomfort as well.

On this new road away from the rotary, you may notice feeling uncomfortable and a little anxious. All new paths (letting go of old habits) create a sense of uncertainty. Treat those feelings as good news. You are breaking new ground. Your tools on this new path are, as always, mindfulness, curiosity and compassion.

Regular practice will make these steps feel more natural and more comfortable. Rather than derailing your day, your BBIMs will become a cue to return to the BodySelf practice. As you do this more and more, you will notice that you spend less time in that old rotary and more time practicing alignment and resourcing.

Right-sizing Your Life

People often think body image is about size and shape. But that doesn't explain why you can wake up with one body image and go to sleep with another. That phenomenon can only be explained by understanding your body image from the inside out. As you begin to practice BodySelfing, you will be in a long-term process of right-sizing your life. Right-sizing is about seeing, acknowledging and resourcing what is happening on the inside, and aligning your life on the outside accordingly. An embodied and aligned life leads to a life that is closer to the right size and shape for you. Ways to Right-Size your life:

- When you feel the pang of wanting to be fitter or tighter, more ripped or less squishy (or whatever might be "wrong" with your body), take the time to listen to how you feel and how your body is responding to what is going on in your life.

- When you no longer expect yourself to do what you don't have energy or desire to do and you practice new boundaries.

- When you honor yourself and show up in relationships as a shape that is your own rather than one that is contorted to fit another person's puzzle piece.

- When you remind yourself of the hierarchy of your own values, and make decisions and choices based on these and not based on a comparison to someone else's.

- When you have the courage to experiment with and lean into what feels right to you, not what you were taught was supposed to feel right.

- When your experience of getting dressed supports you in being you in the world.

Client Spotlight: Values Organized

Gabby was one year into parenting twins she adopted on her own at birth. Though she had done all the reading and purchased every toy and gadget, she was not prepared for how much it changed her life. Her heart had grown bigger, and she loved her new family, but it was challenging to accept a life that left almost no room for who she was before. Her long rides with a cycling group turned into walks pushing a stroller. Her once organized house became a sea of baby-related contraptions.

With the help of her executive coach, she accepted that this was the year to embrace being good enough. Yet she often compared herself to her neighbors with beautiful holiday decor outside their homes, her friends celebrating their long weekend bike rides and the people on her team outselling her in recent months. She developed a habit of stopping what she was doing when she noticed her comparisons became particularly loud and would internally list her values in order of importance: physical and mental health, taking care of and spending time with family, continued (moderate) success at work. When she really tapped into what she had committed to and what she valued in her life, it helped quiet the negative voices clamoring for a tighter butt, a cleaner house and the extra praise at work. She knew that when she looked back on her life, she would be proud of where she directed her energy and wouldn't remember how fit she was or what her living room looked like.

"Transformation includes loss."

Joel Monk

Growth, Grief and the BodySelf

In learning to connect more deeply with our bodies, we will inevitably encounter some grief and loss. Loss is an inevitable aspect of life that is often an embodied experience. We may have losses from long ago that we have not yet fully addressed. We may realize there are certain people or aspects of our life that no longer feel aligned and it can feel helpful to honor the significance of these losses. As we get more connected to ourselves, we may also feel grief for our ideal body and everything that we associated with it. Grief can show up for so many reasons and none of them are wrong. When we cap our capacity for the darker emotions, we are also capping our capacity for the brighter ones as well. Few of us have had role models offering strategies for navigating the grieving process. In addressing grief and loss, we always encourage companionship and guidance through friends, a group, therapy, coaching or spiritual direction.

Client Spotlight: Out-of-Body Experience

Amanda was a highly respected senior manager at her company. She was promoted faster than any of her peers and wound up seeking an executive coach because she felt so much anxiety about the employees she managed. Many of her direct reports were struggling but she couldn't seem to help them improve. She redirected much of this frustration into long hours at work and her fitness regime, which entailed a high-intensity bootcamp. Even when her body was feeling depleted and in need of rest, she would still show up for work and bootcamp.

Amanda's partner had died three years prior, and her sister became ill earlier in the year. The stress, travel and rewards of work and workouts distracted her from feeling the pain of these losses. She had abandoned all her self-care practices and was going from airplane to computer to gym to bed most days.

Amanda recognized that she was in an unsustainable pattern that didn't feel good, but coming out of the pattern was scary. Slowly and with care, she and her coach explored ways to nourish her body rather than abandon it. She looked for a therapist to help her address her grief, put several of her direct reports on performance plans and tiptoed back into her yoga practice. As she became more connected to herself, she was able to set more boundaries at work and create more space to attend to her unprocessed grief.

If we have been chasing a better body image for most of our life, we can feel grief in letting go of that ideal. You may grieve as you shift your relationship with your negative body image and what it promised. After years spent living for a "someday" body, we may fear letting go of this future self and everything that went along with that dream. Know, however, that if we take this difficult step, we can trust that we are trading in "someday" for something else: an authentic connection to ourselves. This alignment is often what we were originally hoping for, we just didn't know how to get there.

Invisible Victories: Championing Ourselves

Most of the successes of the BodySelf journey live outside the traditional glory zone. The words "celebration" and "victory" imply being seen and recognized. There are no awards or medals for choosing curiosity and compassion over self-criticism or for responding directly to your emotional needs instead of trying to change your body. We call these significant moments of progress "Invisible Victories" because no one but you may see them. Honoring our Invisible Victories gives us permission to celebrate our progress, our experiments and our wins even if they are invisible to everyone else. The reality is that some of our most hard-earned wins may only be known to us.

At the core of the Invisible Victory is self-mirroring—where you see yourself in a positive and connected way. Feeling an Invisible Victory is an extension of inside-out training. You are bypassing your body image for validation. Instead of trying to change the body to get something for yourself, with an Invisible Victory you are directly offering warmth, connection and understanding to your insides. To internalize your BodySelf training, look for and find your Invisible Victory each day. In the evenings, you may set aside a quiet moment to review the day, look for an Invisible Victory and fully feel your progress and your connection to your core self.

How do we celebrate Invisible Victories? We are not suggesting lavish parties or spraying champagne in the air (although that sounds fun and should not be out of the question!) We are talking about taking the time and attention to acknowledge, witness and honor new choices and our small and large wins. It could be as simple as recognizing it yourself or sharing it with a trusted friend. You could write yourself a card and mail it to your own address. You could do a dance or buy yourself something nice. You could literally pat yourself on the back or pump your fist in the air. The gesture itself is not important—it is the intentionality behind it. Practice mirroring yourself; give yourself the experience of being seen and celebrated.

Invisible Victory examples:
- Directly addressing an issue instead of blaming your body—taking a new step on the BodySelf Rotary.
- Buying the bigger pant size rather than saying you will lose weight to fit into the ones you have.

- Being more accepting and less critical when you don't exercise in your usual way when historically that was not possible.
- Tolerating the discomfort of declining an event you feel you "should" go to but you know will leave you feeling lousy given who will be there.
- Speaking up in a meeting where you historically are quiet.
- Allowing yourself to feel the discomfort of an interaction and turning to a compassionate support to vent or process when you usually push such feelings away.

Exercise 10.2 Invisible Victories

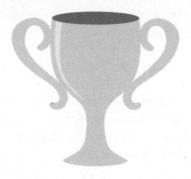

This Invisible Victory is awarded to _____ *for*

_____

What strengths did it require from you?

_____

_____

What growth edge did you push?

_____

_____

What was hard about it?

_____

_____

What felt good about it?

_____

_____

What are you proud of?

_____

_____

Who would you like to share this accomplishment with?

_____

_____

Mindset Check-in

Remember capturing your body image mindset in Chapter 1? Now that you have done the brave work of getting curious, translating, decoding, rerouting and experimenting, let's do that exercise again and see what has changed.

What I believe to be true about my body image is:

_____

_____

The way this makes me feel is:

_____

_____

The way this makes me act is:

_____

_____

The BodySelf skills I want to focus on most are:

_____

_____

Looking ahead on my body image journey I am most curious about:

_____

_____

"Life is not what you alone make it. Life is the input of everyone who touched your life and every experience that entered it. We are all part of one another."

Yuri Kochiyama

You Are Not Alone

Now you are finishing this book and heading off to practice those ideas that resonated the most with you. Maybe this feels exciting or maybe it seems daunting, or perhaps both. As you finish this book, let's take a moment with your body and with your immediate contact with the book—your hands. Look down at your hands as they hold this book. Really look at their color, their shape, their size. Know that there are other people, with hands of the same and different sizes and shapes and colors, holding this book on this page and wondering the very same thing. Imagine these hands and these people for a moment. Imagine wanting them to have more peace in their body and less self-hate in their mind. Imagine that the ways you practice your BodySelf tools will help them. And imagine the ways they practice will help you. You are not alone.

Bless all that is right-sizing within you.

Bless the grief, the discomfort, the emerging ...
Bless your growls, your groans and your sighs
as you birth this next version of yourself.

Bless the tussle with the new and the old as
you vacillate between falling in love with
yourself and the nasty snarl of self-hatred.

Bless you as you journey towards what fits
on the inside, on the outside and the spaces in between.

Bless the unique shape of you
And your right to inhabit this shape.

To not fight or damage or hate it.

Bless the unique shape of you.

Appendix
Internal Family Systems (IFS)

Many teachings and approaches have informed this book, yet none as strongly as the Internal Family Systems model developed by Richard Schwartz.* Internal Family Systems has enriched our work both personally and professionally. While we created the BodySelf approach before we knew IFS existed, IFS has offered more nuance to our understanding of how and why our negative body image may have stepped in to try to help us. IFS is complementary to the BodySelf, as it also beautifully encourages an internal dialogue with aspects of ourselves—which is what we are all about! If you have been introduced to IFS in your own personal therapy or use it as a practitioner, we want to amplify your ability to incorporate body image work into your IFS practice.

IFS and Negative Body Image

As we have emphasized throughout this book, body image is a topic people often shy away from. It is loaded, intimate and also universal. People often fear saying the wrong thing, feeling awkward or overstepping boundaries. If you are working within an IFS framework, you can lean into body image-related topics and treat these body image *parts* the way you would any other *protector parts*. We encourage you to see body image-related beliefs and patterns as well-intentioned *protectors* and with deep compassion and become curious about how these *parts* are trying to serve the greater system. In the following sections, we offer a translation of sorts: using IFS language for some of the BodySelf concepts that have been presented throughout this book.

---

* For those of you who are unfamiliar with Internal Family Systems, it is a form of psychotherapy that conceptualizes that we are each born with our own unique set of "parts," aspects of our true nature, that operate within us like an "internal family." The IFS model teaches that along with our various "parts," we all have an inner wisdom and wholeness at our core, what they call "Self." We are all born with "Self" energy and it can't be diminished, regardless of what we have been through. Ideally, "Self" leads our system and we move through the world and make decisions from this grounded, connected state. However, we all have "parts" that are impacted by our experiences, particularly when we are young, and these parts move into more exaggerated roles in order to help us adapt to our environment when we may not have had other resources or support. These parts may continue to use these same extreme strategies over time, not realizing that we have developed other tools. Through compassion and curiosity, IFS offers a method of building relationships with these extreme parts so that our system can come back into balance and we can be more "Self" led. The goal is never to eliminate parts but to help them heal so that rather than overtaking our system, they become assets to it, allowing "Self" to naturally lead the way. If you are interested to learn more about IFS, check out ifs-institute.com.

"When you first meet me, you might meet my bodyguard."

Anne Lamott

Body Image "Parts"

The BodySelf and IFS view our critical thoughts and beliefs about our bodies as inner warriors who have been loyal and committed to our protection. Body image *parts* can show up in many ways, though most often as managers who compare, criticize or push us to do or not do things, often in the service of achieving greater safety or connection. Much like the way we befriended our beloved Fat Temp and Crazy Raisin all those years ago, IFS invites us to identify our various parts and to build relationships with them. Critical body image *parts* often have held a lifelong belief that being in a certain body will give us access to something we are longing for. These *parts* may have come to believe that letting go of our "body goal" would mean losing hope for whatever that idealized body offers. By listening with compassion and curiosity to what our critical body image *parts* really want for us, we can start working collaboratively with these parts and offer them other resources and strategies to achieve what they so desperately want for us. One of the tenets of IFS that we find so powerful is actively offering gratitude to our *parts* for their efforts. When we turn towards our *parts* and acknowledge the ways that they have been working so hard on our behalf, something shifts. These protective *parts* become more open to the idea of dialing down their intensity and considering a more collaborative relationship when they feel understood.

Here is an example of a seemingly critical body image *part* working hard in challenging circumstances, and how with curiosity and compassion, parts can become less extreme and more in balance.

Client Spotlight: Mean Coach

Abby couldn't recall a time when she *didn't* have a critical voice telling her that she needed to be stronger and fitter. She experienced this *part* much like the mean coach on the show *Glee*—wearing an Adidas tracksuit, with a whistle around her neck, pacing back and forth on the sidelines. Abby's "Mean Coach" screamed at her constantly, telling her that she wasn't moving her body enough and demanding a stronger commitment to exercise. "Mean Coach's" demands for Abby to improve her fitness overrode Abby's natural desire for breaks, time off and rest. Abby may have felt like a nap but her "Mean Coach" would demand a long run. For most of Abby's life, this part had left her feeling sad, exhausted and beaten down. Yet once Abby was able to see her "Mean Coach" as a *part* of her, and bring more curiosity to her "Mean Coach's" intentions, she was able to see how hard this part had been working on her behalf.

Abby's role in her family was complex and unrewarding. Both her father and brother had untreated bipolar disorder and refused any sort of mental health treatment. Her mom saw Abby as her primary support, confiding in and burdening Abby with her overwhelm and grief. Abby's family assumed that because she was such a competent student and stand-out athlete, that she could manage herself *and* help caretake the household.

Abby's "Mean Coach," while nasty in her approach, was doing everything she could to try to help her navigate her home life. First, "Mean Coach" directed Abby's attention toward accomplishments that were achievable, offering Abby hope and a sense of impact in an environment that felt bleak. "Mean Coach" was also trying to create the boundaries with her family that felt impossible for Abby to set on her own by demanding a highly regimented exercise schedule. "Mean Coach" knew that Abby's family drew pride from her athletic successes and would let her take time away from the household chaos to train. "Mean Coach's" primary goal was to make Abby a star athlete, to help her feel differentiated from her family. Abby had so little room for her own dreams and this part offered her promise that her life could be different and that she deserved to have more agency and possibility in her life ahead.

Our *parts'* intentions are always good. "Mean Coach" only wanted Abby to feel more empowered and less burdened. Reflecting back, Abby was in awe of all of the ways that her "Mean Coach" had been trying to protect her over the years. As Abby came to see her "Mean Coach" with understanding and even respect, "Mean Coach" started to soften. As Abby created a more collaborative relationship with her "Mean Coach," she could see that there were times where she needed this part's essence (an upcoming half marathon) but that she had many other tools to support her in managing her life and the ongoing challenges of her family's issues.

Here is an example of what can be uncovered when a part of us experiences change or loss.

Client Spotlight: Fashionista

As an interior designer and an artist, Kaya had always enjoyed expressing herself through fashion and she called this creative part of herself "Fashionista." She appreciated the role that fashion played in her life, but it wasn't until the COVID lockdown of 2020 that this *part's* job fully revealed its function. Because everyone was working from home during the Pandemic, Kaya's "Fashionista" part wasn't able to express itself or be "seen" in the ways that she had come to rely on. Without the opportunity to show off her unique style and artistic eye, she felt invisible, unmoored and depressed.

Kaya knew the lockdown was hard on everyone in different ways, but she was perplexed about why her mood had sunk so dramatically and wanted to understand why. With more inquiry, Kaya was able to locate a *part* she was less familiar with that longed for a certain kind of recognition and connection. As Kaya got to know this *part*, she discovered that this young *part* was a product of the extensive time she had spent with her best friend Olivia growing up, often to escape the lack of emotional safety in her own home. Olivia's home was warm and inviting and her family was close-knit, in contrast to Kaya's which was chaotic, with parents who were distracted and overwhelmed. Olivia's mom was a stylist and loved helping her kids find their own unique sense of style. Olivia and her mom loved to shop together and they often took Kaya along. Kaya felt so much joy on these adventures and the more Olivia and her mom encouraged Kaya to express herself through her clothing, the more her confidence grew.

Kaya's "Fashionista" *part* evolved over time as a way to both be creative and express herself but she didn't realize the behind-the-scenes role it had played until it was taken away. It wasn't until "Fashionista" lost the access to express herself creatively and be celebrated for her unique style that Kaya's younger *part* was exposed and her deeper longings to feel safe and seen revealed themselves. This younger *part*'s desire for stability and connection had become conflated with having style and looking "put together," much like Olivia's family. Kaya's young *part* believed that fashion was the gateway to security and support. It was humbling and powerful for Kaya to discover the layers of herself that her "Fashionista" *part* was tending to. While the isolation of the pandemic was a very painful time, Kaya was grateful to discover a deeper level of healing she didn't know she needed.

The following is an example of a protector *part* using comparison as a way to feel a sense of acceptance.

Client Spotlight: Comparing as Currency

Ella had a *part* that habitually compared her body to others and when she got to graduate school, this *part* became even more pronounced. She had always been acutely aware of other people's bodies relative to her own, but when she entered the program, she found herself scanning every room, analyzing the size and appearance of all of her peers. By identifying and bringing curiosity to this "Comparing" *part*, she was able to learn more about when it came to be and how it was trying to help. The *part* had developed when she was an adolescent, growing up in a family culture that was highly critical and vocal about other people's size and appearance. Both her parents and extended family were in constant dialogue about how others looked, often labeling them with cruel words if they didn't dress in a flattering way and/or have a certain body size that they deemed ideal. She didn't get any mirroring from her family, so she harnessed the measuring tool she saw them using most often. Her "Comparing" *part* had internalized her family's messages and believed it was vital to look "put together," have the "right" body and not stand out in order to be accepted and find success.

As an adult, Ella knew her value went far beyond appearance, yet her *part* used comparison as a way to steady her when her sense of place, value or belonging was in question — which was most new experiences! Because she had not been seen or anchored well in her early years, her "Comparing" *part* often stepped in to orient her when things felt uncertain or unknown.

Once Ella understood how this *part* came to be and how it was trying to help her transition to graduate school, she was able to recognize that at this stage of her life, she could build alternative ways to ground and support herself. She had compassion for how invisible she had felt in her family and how her size and appearance had become the controllables she could focus on when things felt new and uncomfortable. Ella let her "Comparing" *part* know how much she appreciated all the ways it had tried to protect and support her growing up and was able to help this part trust that Ella had access to other resources for these big life transitions.

We have both been so powerfully impacted by IFS. If you have an existing relationship with IFS and are interested in using it to help yourself or your clients feel more comfortable working with body image, we encourage you to bring the same curiosity and compassion towards body image-related parts as any other parts you work with.

> *"IFS is a way of empowering ourselves to be our own healer, and to trust our own inner wisdom."*
>
> Richard Schwartz

BodySelf Glossary

Bad Body Image Moment (BBIM): A BodySelf nickname for when our negative body image spikes.

BodySelf (noun): An approach and practice that explores how negative body image beliefs are shaped by our environment, history, culture and the context of the present moment. It is a framework to investigate and heal negative body image through a lens of curiosity and compassion. *Have you heard about that cool new book about how to get in touch with your BodySelf?*

BodySelf (verb): The act of exploring, relating to and healing one's negative body image through a framework of curiosity and compassion. *You sound awfully self-critical, you might want to do some BodySelfing.*

Embodiment: The experience of being present *inside* our body, the practice of being more present to our internal experience.

Finding alignment: The process of listening for our resonance to identify what in the outside world feels in agreement with our body. Finding alignment is the opposite of shapeshifting. It's using your unique body cues to find your inner resonance.

Interoception: The collection of senses providing us information about the internal state of our body.

Resonance: The felt sense that signals that our body is in agreement with external stimuli.

Resourcing: Listening and responding to the messages our body is giving us about what we may need or want.

Shapeshifting: An adaptation that involves "reshaping ourselves" (our behaviors and how we present ourselves) to improve the dynamics in our relationships. Shapeshifting initially plays out emotionally as we try to adapt to the dynamics around us and over time these patterns can evolve into changing our *literal* shape in order to shift a relational outcome.

For additional downloadable copies of some of the most commonly used exercises in the book and a BodySelf parents handout visit our website: **www.thebodyself.com**.

Acknowledgments

This book was a labor of love. Many authors talk about books writing themselves and to us, it felt like this book did just that. We set out to self-publish a compilation of our workshop's greatest hits but chapters kept having babies and it ended up being far more comprehensive than we ever imagined. It helped us expand our knowledge and definition of what we mean by the BodySelf and deepen our conviction that strategies for working with negative body image are crucial to building greater connection with ourselves. This book made us into better writers and clinicians. We want to thank "Body Image Inside Out" for being our teacher in ways we are still discovering. We couldn't have written this book without EVERY SINGLE BBIM we have had along the way. Each one taught us more about ourselves and challenged us to live our work. While Fat Temp and Crazy Raisin are the origin story, our clients are the true heroes whose bravery showed us the power of the BodySelf approach through their stories of transformation.

Our Gratitude

Together we want to thank Michael Otto, whose experience and gifted editing eye helped this book become more clear and confident in its voice and offering. We are grateful to Jim for being our spelling and punctuation wizard, helping us comb through our most tangled sentences and being so deeply committed to co-creating our perfect cover palette. Natalie, thank you for your encouragement, deep understanding of the book's message and extraordinary editing that got us over heartbreak hill. Sarah, we are forever grateful for your coaching that catapulted our publishing acumen from novice to educated and guided us to our publishing home. We want to thank Rachel and Megan and the team at Sheldon for believing in our work. Chloe, your kindness and patience was so appreciated. Thank you Jenni Bonito, our endlessly patient and talented graphic designer, and Mallory, thank you for sharing your super powers. Robin, there are no words for your magic. And we want to thank one another—without our keen powers of self-awareness, our resilience and our courage we would not have created the BodySelf nor gotten the book over the finish line. We also want to thank the gnomes who wrote the sentences and paragraphs that neither of us remember writing and insist on giving the other person credit for.

Deb's Gratitude

Jim, thank you for your unending love and support through every step of this process. Your curiosity, patience and cooking skills kept me going. I also want to express my deep love and appreciation to my wise and loving therapists and supervisors who have had such a huge impact on me over the years … pieces of all of you are in this book. Ellen #1, Laura, Justin, Rachel, Ellen #2, Cheryl, Rheta and especially Julia and Jeanne, for reminding me that my clients and I have everything we need inside us to heal. And my gifted body workers who helped put my body back together again more times than I can count. I feel such love, awe and gratitude for my parents, my brother Josh and my Cherow cousins, who have taught me so much about the power of asking great questions and listening with love. I treasure my compassionate, loving and supportive friends who cheered me on: Anne, Alison, Cara, CJ, Davey, Eryn, Jenny, Maddie, Marci, Nanny G, Natalie, Roger and Roz. And of course my furry soulmates, Bella and Soleil.

Whitney's Gratitude

Thank you to Michael Otto the husband—without the foundation our relationship gives me, I wouldn't have been able to show up to all the emotional and editorial challenges writing this book required. I am grateful to Judy, Bill, Steph, Barti and Erin, who skillfully and lovingly held spaces for me to heal into being comfortable in my own skin. Thank you Summer and West for rolling your eyes whenever I mentioned Chapter 4, enduring my weekends away and grumpiness from late-night writing bursts. You both inspire me to be the truest, most loving and courageous version of myself I can be—which fueled the writing of this book. Thank you to my encouraging friends who sent flowers when I hit deadlines, and listened to a million book status updates, and gently asked, "Is it done yet?"

Index